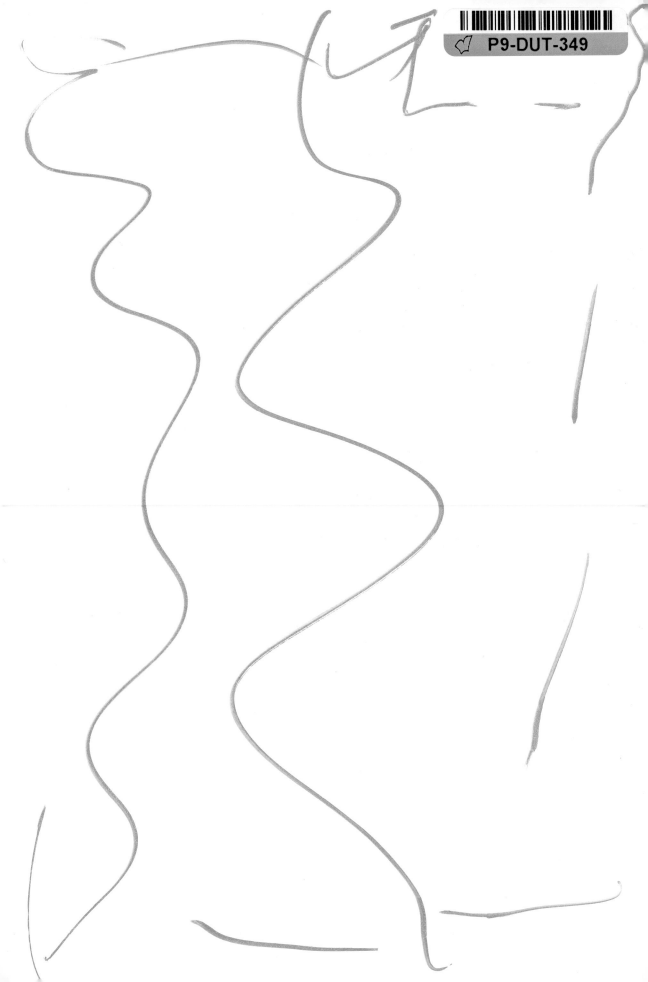

The Child with Down's Syndrome

(Mongolism)

Causes, Characteristics and Acceptance

**FOR PARENTS, PHYSICIANS
AND PERSONS CONCERNED
WITH HIS EDUCATION AND CARE**

DAVID W. SMITH, M.D. *and* ANN ASPER WILSON

Dysmorphology Unit,
Department of Pediatrics,
University of Washington Medical School,
Seattle, Washington

Formerly, Dysmorphology Unit,
Department of Pediatrics
University of Washington Medical School
Seattle, Washington

W. B. SAUNDERS COMPANY
Philadelphia   London   Toronto
Mexico City   Rio de Janeiro   Sydney   Tokyo

W. B. Saunders Company: West Washington Square
Philadelphia, PA   19105

1 St. Anne's Road
Eastbourne, East Sussex BN21 3UN, England

1 Goldthorne Avenue
Toronto, Ontario M8Z 5T9, Canada

Apartado 26370—Cedro 512
Mexico 4, D.F., Mexico

Rua Coronel Cabrita, 8
Sao Cristovao Caixa Postal 21176
Rio de Janeiro, Brazil

9 Waltham Street
Artarmon, N.S.W. 2064, Australia

Ichibancho, Central Bldg., 22-1 Ichibancho
Chiyoda-Ku, Tokyo 102, Japan

Listed here is the latest translated edition of this book together
with the language of the translation and the publisher.

French (1st Edition)—Editions du Centurion, Paris, France

Japanese (1st Edition)—Gakuen Sha Ltd.

Spanish (1st Edition)—Editorial Medica Panamericana, Buenos Aires, Argentina

The Child with Down's Syndrome   ISBN   0-7216-8420-3

Print No.:   18   17   16   15   14   13   12

To
Down's syndrome children
and their parents

Acknowledgments

Parents: The authors wish to acknowledge and thank the numerous parents whose shared experiences and thoughts aided in the development of this book, especially those who contributed to the final chapter: Mr. and Mrs. Eugene Ballard, Mr. and Mrs. Spencer Hill, Mr. and Mrs. Robert Otteson, Mr. and Mrs. Lloyd Reichel, and Mr. and Mrs. Glen L. Schultz.

Memorial: The Charles Duncan Woodside Memorial Fund provided for medical illustration and photography, which greatly enhanced the educational value of this book. Charles, the son of Dr. and Mrs. Chester W. Woodside, died in infancy of complications of Down's syndrome. The authors sincerely hope this book will be at least a partially fitting tribute to the memory of Charles, by helping the parents of other children with Down's syndrome.

Photography: Mr. Daniel L. Gluck, free-lance photographer, is most gratefully acknowledged as the photographer for most of the pictures in the photo album section of this book. We also thank the University of Washington Department of Medical Photography for its contributions.

Illustrations: Mrs. Phyllis Wood of the University of Washington Department of Medical Illustration prepared most of the illustrations.

Secretaries: Mrs. Mary Pearlman and Mrs. Mary Ann Harvey have been most helpful in the development of this book.

Research Librarian: Mrs. Lyle Harrah was extremely helpful in researching the literature for this book.

Rainier School: Dr. Albert Reichert, Superintendent of Ranier School, and many others at the school were most helpful in providing ideas and material for this book. Some of the pictures in the photo album section provide obvious evidence of the exemplary nature and attitude of this state institution for the mentally deficient.

University of Washington Experimental Education Unit: Acknowledgment is made to the Experimental Education Unit of the Child Development and Mental Retardation Center, which provides a program for young Down's syndrome children and their families. This is a part of the Model Preschool Center for Handicapped Children, a project directed by Dr. Alice H. Hayden, Associate Director of the Unit. Mrs. Valentine Dmitriev, coordinator of the program for the Down's syndrome children, was especially helpful. Many of the photo album pictures attest to the enrichment which this program is providing for these young children with Down's syndrome.

Others: The help of Mr. and Mrs. David DeNini, who developed the group home shown in the photo album, is gratefully acknowledged. We wish to thank Mr. Bradley Gong for the actual chromosome preparations shown in Chapter 1.

Funding: This book was developed in the Dysmorphology Unit, a unit dedicated to teaching, service, and research about problems of malformation. The unit derives its major financial support from the Department of Health, Education and Welfare (MCHS and HSMA, Project 913) and partial support from The National Foundation.

Contents

vii

3

4

Introduction

Every baby, with or without Down's syndrome, is a unique person. He will grow up having his own smile, his own laugh, his own distinctive habits, likes, and dislikes. The development of his personality and of his physical and mental being will be determined by inherited genetic factors combined with cultural and environmental influences. Blended together, they create a person unlike any other person born before or afterward. All these factors make up a potential, a potential that can be realized in time with growth and good health, with education and training, with a warm and happy environment. It is a parent's challenge to seek out his child's capabilities and areas of possible development, to understand his limitations, both physical and mental, and to provide him with opportunities to grow and learn as he is able.

The child with Down's syndrome, like other children, has a potential, but it is a limited one. It is limited even before the time of birth, from the very beginning of the mother's pregnancy. For, in the earliest stages of growth in the mother's uterus, the developing individual with Down's syndrome carries a genetic imbalance; that is, by a simple mistake he has an extra set of genes on an extra chromosome. This extra one is added to the usual number of 46 chromosomes which are found in every cell in his body. It is usually a perfectly normal chromosome, but the extra set of genes creates a fundamental genetic imbalance. This genetic imbalance causes the alterations of growth and development seen in the child with Down's syndrome, and it is the most important factor in determining what his potential will be.

Down's syndrome is the most common serious problem in development seen in a newborn. It occurs more frequently than any other specific kind of mental deficiency or any single error in early development such as

1

cleft lip or clubfoot. On the average, one in 640 babies has Down's syndrome; for young mothers the risk of having an affected child is low, but the risk increases progressively with the mother's age. In 1967, it was estimated that of the 3.5 million babies born in the United States, more than 5,000 had Down's syndrome. Down's syndrome can occur in any family. Every race and social class has produced children with Down's syndrome. Because of this universality, doctors have acquired considerable knowledge about how the syndrome affects children and what they will be like as they grow up. The genetic cause of Down's syndrome, however, was not understood until 1959. This new knowledge now enables doctors to counsel parents more accurately about the risk of recurrence. This book presents information about the genetic causes of Down's syndrome and describes the features of the condition that are common to most children who have it. Understanding some of the factors that will influence the life and the future growth of their child will, we hope, provide parents with a better basis for making *their own* decisions concerning the baby's future and the well-being of the family.

A word is necessary regarding the term "Down's syndrome." Langdon Down was an English physician who in 1866 described the features of children with this syndrome. "Syndrome," in this context, means a recognizable *pattern* of altered development. Some people may feel "Down's syndrome" is a rather stuffy, scientific name for the common age-old problem of "mongolism." But there are good reasons why "mongolism" deserves a new name and a fresh approach. There are few physical or mental conditions that are burdened with as many misconceptions as is "mongolism." The very phrase "mongoloid child" suggests a racial or physical relation to an Oriental people that is unsubstantiated. In the past "mongoloids" were often believed to be hopelessly retarded and unmanageable, and were often denied the understanding and simple training all children deserve. Today our knowledge about the genetic and physical aspects of the syndrome and a new resolve to tackle the problems of mental deficiency have given children with Down's syndrome a somewhat brighter future. Much of this new information, particularly about the causes of Down's syndrome, we will present here.

This book is addressed primarily to parents as a guide to understanding what their child will be like and how he came to have Down's syndrome. We hope, too, that others who work with these children will find it useful. Many physicians may be able to employ it in counseling parents. Teachers and social workers also may find it useful as a general reference about the origins and nature of the syndrome.

REFERENCE

Down, J. L.: Observations on ethnic classifications. *London Hospital Reports* 3:259–262, 1866.

1

How Did It Happen? The Genetic Causes and Risks of Down's Syndrome

A baby is born, and after a thorough examination the doctor concludes that he has Down's syndrome. What does that mean? How did it happen, and when? Could it happen again to another child in the same family, as yet unborn? Can it be prevented in future pregnancies?

The Cause

First of all, it is reassuring to know that nothing "went wrong" during those 9 months of the mother's pregnancy. Nothing she ate, or took as medication, no activity or emotional experience could have caused Down's syndrome. The event that produced Down's syndrome in the baby happened before or at about the time the pregnancy began. It happened in the development of the egg or sperm or shortly after they came together at conception. The event was a mistake that altered the correct number of chromosomes to be found in each cell of the new growing baby. A child born with Down's syndrome has an extra chromosome in every cell in his body. It is this extra chromosome which produces the alterations in physical and mental development we find in Down's syndrome.

Chromosomes and Development

Chromosomes are tiny structures found in the nucleus of every cell in the body. There are 46 chromosomes, or 23 matching pairs, in each normal cell. Each pair is designated with a number, from 1 to 22; the twenty-third pair is the sex chromosome pair. The chromosomes of a normal girl are shown in Figure 1. A child with Down's syndrome usually has 47

NORMAL GIRL

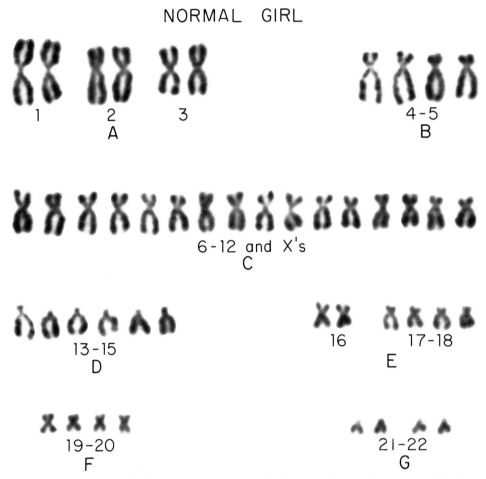

Figure 1.   The chromosomes of a normal girl, cut out from a photomicrograph of one cell just before its division. The chromosomes are arranged according to their size and shape. Some of the pairs can be distinguished, but many cannot; hence the letter groupings. The number 21 pair is in the G group.

chromosomes, with one extra chromosome 21 added to the normal number 21 chromosome pair. This is called *trisomy 21*. The chromosomes of a girl with Down's syndrome are shown in Figure 2.

A chromosome is made up of thousands of "genes." This genetic material is critical to an individual's growth and development, for the genes are like a computer, programming the code the body uses to develop and function. The genes found on one chromosome work in conjunction with the similar genes on its partner chromosome. In order for them to work properly they must be normal, "good" genes. An altered gene may program the wrong code, thus producing an alteration in development. A child with trisomy 21 has normal, "good" genes on his three number 21 chromosomes. It is important also that each gene balance harmoniously with its matching gene on the partner chromosome. Because there are three sets of number 21 genes in a child with Down's syndrome, and not the usual two, the genetic balance is upset, and thus alterations in development are produced.

A normal child receives 46 chromosomes from his parents. Twenty-three, one chromosome from each pair, come from the mother, in the egg. Twenty-three, the other "matching" chromosomes of each pair, come from the father, in the sperm. When the sperm fertilizes the egg, the 46 chromosomes come together to make up the baby's own unique set of 23 pairs in the beginning cell.

The fertilized egg, originally a single cell, grows by a process of cell division; that is, it divides into two identical cells, these divide into four, the four into eight, and on and on. As the cells divide, they change and organize to form tissues and organs. Every time a cell divides to become two cells, the chromosomes must divide also. Between cell divisions each chromosome makes an exact copy (replicate) of itself which remains attached at a juncture point called the centromere. With cell division, the identical chromosomes are separated at at the juncture point, one going into each new cell. Each new cell then has an identical complete set of 46 chromosomes. These processes are illustrated in Figure 3. The normal situation of conception and early cell divisions is illustrated in Figure 4. showing only the number 21 chromosomes.

Faulty Chromosome Distribution Leading to 21 Trisomy Down's Syndrome

It is at the time of cell division, when the chromosomes must accurately distribute themselves, that the problem that causes trisomy 21 arises. What happens, very simply, is a mistake in chromosome distribution. One of the two new cells receives an extra number 21 chromosome, and the other new cell lacks one. All the other chromosome pairs distribute correctly—only the number 21 pair does not. Many, many cell divisions take place during the growth of the baby and throughout life. A mistake in chromosome distribution can occur in any one of them. The severity of its effects on development depends on the timing of the particular cell division in which the mistake occurs. The earlier it is, and thus the fewer cells there are, the more significant the consequences, since all cells deriving from a 21 trisomy cell will also be 21 trisomic.

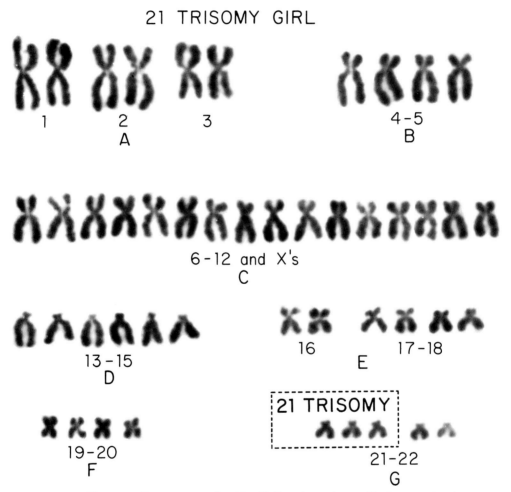

21 TRISOMY GIRL

Figure 2. Chromosomes of a girl with Down's syndrome. She has an extra chromosome 21; this is called trisomy 21.

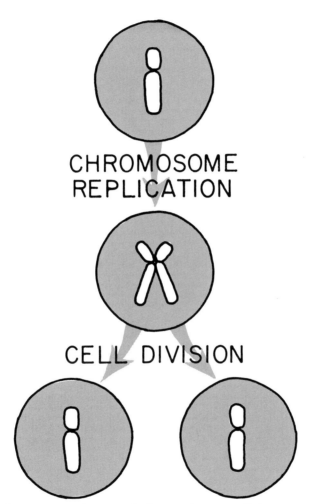

Figure 3. In chromosome replication, which occurs between cell divisions, each chromosome doubles. At cell division the chromosomes separate at the juncture point (centromere) and each new (daughter) cell receives an identical chromosome complement. This is illustrated for just one chromosome.

NORMAL DEVELOPMENT

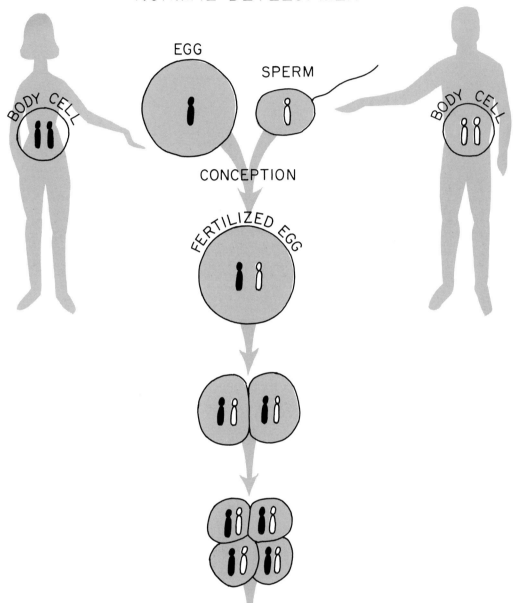

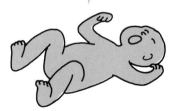

Figure 4. Normal distribution of chromosome number 21, with one of each pair going to the egg or sperm, so that upon combination of egg and sperm there is a pair of each chromosome. This genetically balanced situation leads toward the development of a normal baby.

DOWN'S SYNDROME

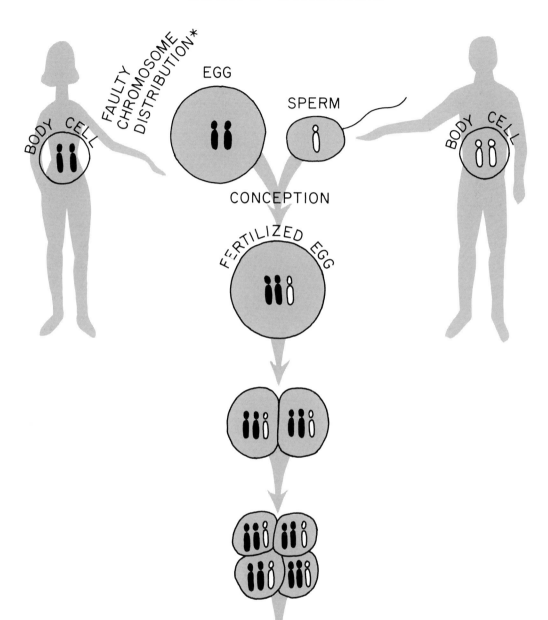

DEVELOPMENT TOWARD A BABY WITH DOWN'S SYNDROME

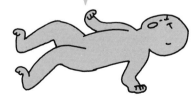

Figure 5.   Faulty chromosome distribution to the egg (or sperm) can lead to 21 trisomy in the fertilized egg. All subsequent cells have this genetic imbalance, which results in the alterations in development known as Down's syndrome.

DOWN'S SYNDROME

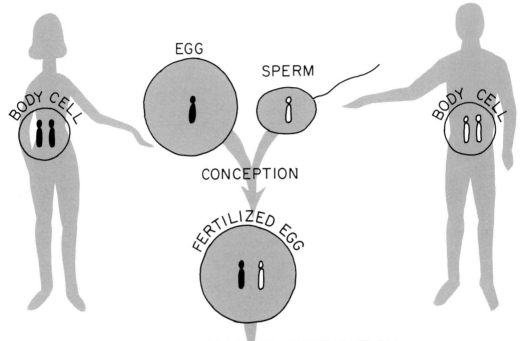

CONCEPTION

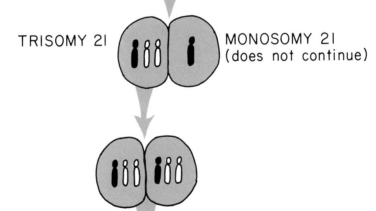

FAULTY CHROMOSOME DISTRIBUTION

TRISOMY 21   MONOSOMY 21
(does not continue)

DEVELOPMENT TOWARD A BABY WITH DOWN'S SYNDROME

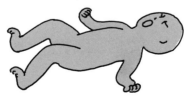

Figure 6.   Faulty distribution of a 21 chromosome in the first cell division of the fertilized egg, leading to 21 trisomy and a baby with Down's syndrome.

DOWN'S SYNDROME (mosaic)

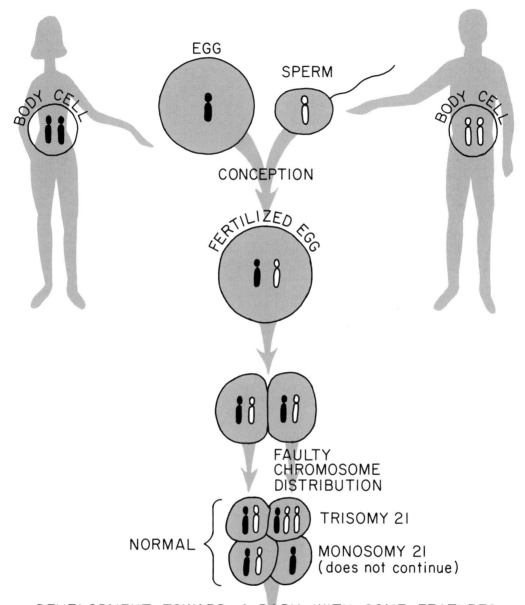

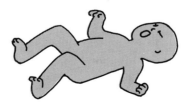

Figure 7. If faulty 21 chromosome distribution occurs in the second cell division, some of the baby's cells will be normal, and some will be 21 trisomic. This is called 21 trisomy/normal mosaicism. Such babies may show partial features of Down's syndrome.

The great majority of children with Down's syndrome have a full trisomy 21; that is, three number 21 chromosomes are present in every cell. In this situation, the timing of the fault in chromosome distribution can probably be placed either in the development of the egg or the sperm, or in the first cell division of the fertilized egg. It is usually impossible to tell which was the case for a specific child.

A mistake in chromosome distribution can occur in the development of an egg or a sperm, because as each forms it goes through several cell divisions. In the beginning, the cells that will become egg or sperm have the parent's 46 chromosomes. In a type of division unique to sex cells, however, the chromosomes distribute so that each egg-to-be or sperm-to-be receives only one chromosome from each pair, or 23 in all. If the number 21 chromosomes do not distribute correctly and both go to one cell, the resultant egg or sperm will carry an extra number 21 chromosome. When it combines with the other parent's egg or sperm, the resulting fertilized egg will have three number 21 chromosomes and will therefore be destined to develop into a child having Down's syndrome. This is conceptualized in Figure 5.

The second possibility is that both the egg and the sperm are normal, but in the very first cell division of the fertilized egg the number 21 chromosomes do not distribute correctly. One new cell receives three number 21 chromosomes (21 trisomy) and the other receives only one. A cell with only one number 21 chromosome cannot function properly and soon dies. The one with trisomy 21 will continue to multiply, and all the cells in the growing baby will have the extra number 21 chromosome. The baby will thus have a full trisomy 21 and consequently Down's syndrome. This is shown in Figure 6.

In about 4 per cent of children with Down's syndrome, distribution mistakes occur in the second, or possibly third, division of the new developing individual. As a result, some of the cells are normal and some have the trisomy 21. This admixture is called 21 trisomy/normal mosaicism, and is depicted in Figure 7. Because a baby who is a 21 trisomy/normal mosaic has a normal chromosome complement in some of his cells, he may have fewer of the physical characteristics and better mental performance than Down's syndrome children with 21 trisomy in all cells. Mosaicism can generally be determined by chromosome studies.

Translocation 21 Trisomy, an Unusual Cause for Down's Syndrome

In an additional 4 per cent of children with Down's syndrome the extra number 21 chromosome has broken and its long arm is attached to the broken end of another chromosome. This rearrangement of two chromosomes is called a translocation, as shown in Figure 8. Such a translocation chromosome may be made up of a rearrangement of a number 14 chromosome and a 21 chromosome, as one example. With a pair of normal 21 chromosomes plus this extra long arm of 21 chromosome, the effect of the extra set of 21 genes is Down's syndrome. Though unusual, the translocation 21 trisomy can be distinguished from the full 21 trisomy only by chromosome studies. It deserves mention because it is possible that, in about one-third of translocation 21 trisomy cases, one of the parents who is normal physically and mentally can be a genetically balanced carrier of the translocation chromosome. The balanced translocation carrier parent does not have the third number 21 chromosome, but one of his two number 21 chromosomes is attached to another chromosome so that he has a total of only 45 chromosomes. This attachment does not alter the normal balance and function of his genes, and hence such a translocation carrier parent is normal in both appearance and intelligence. The balanced translocation carrier situation is depicted in Figure 8. In the development of the egg or sperm from a translocation carrier parent, the translocation chromosome may be distributed to a cell along with the normal number 21 chromosome, so that the resulting egg or sperm has two sets of number 21 chromosome genes. When it joins a normal egg or sperm from the other parent, the fertilized egg will have three sets of number 21 chromosome genes.

The risk of a balanced translocation carrier parent having a child with Down's syndrome varies with the type of translocation. The following are the risks for the more common types: If the mother is the translocation carrier, her risk of having a child with Down's syndrome is believed to be 10 per cent or higher with each pregnancy. If the father is a translocation carrier the risk runs about 2 per cent or higher. Why the difference? It would seem that a sperm carrying the chromosome imbalance is less likely to be the first one to arrive and fertilize the egg, whereas this type of selection does not exist for the egg.

Translocation 21 trisomy type of Down's syndrome is relatively unusual. It is more frequent, however, among children with Down's syndrome born to young parents, accounting for about 6 per cent of such cases. Thus it is often advisable for babies with Down's syndrome born to mothers under 30 years of age to have a chromosome analysis to exclude the possibility of the translocation type of Down's syndrome. If the baby has a translocation chromosome, the parents should then have a chromosome study to determine whether either is a balanced translocation carrier. Overall, the general chance that one of young parents of a child with Down's syndrome will be found to be a translocation carrier is only about 2 per cent.

HOW CHROMOSOME STUDIES ARE DONE.   Some hospitals are now equipped to do chromosome studies. A small amount of blood is taken and the white blood cells are grown for several days until there are a large number of dividing cells. The cells are chemically treated to stop their growth at the point of cell division. The cells are then disrupted so that the chromosomes spread out. The chromosomes are placed on a glass slide, stained, and observed through the microscope. Photographs are made, and the individual chromosomes are cut out and arranged in accordance with their size and the position of the juncture point, or so-called centromere, of the chromosome. A picture of chromosomes arranged in their proper order is called a karyotype (see Figures 1, 2, and 9).

If a baby who is suspected of having Down's syndrome has 47, not 46, chromosomes, and the extra one compares with the 21-size chromosomes, it can be assumed that the baby has a full trisomy 21. In a case such as this it is generally not necessary to study the parents' chromosomes. If the baby has a translocation chromosome, the number of chromosomes will

Formation of a Translocation Chromosome

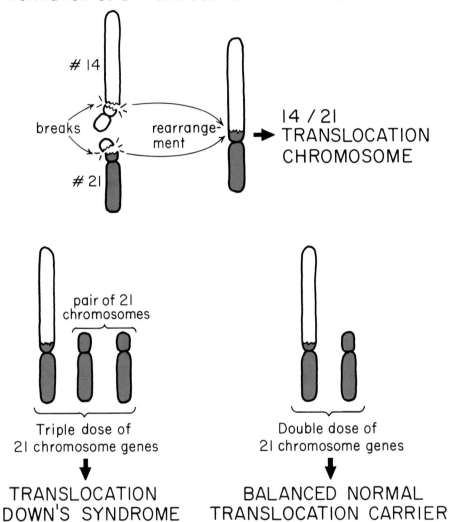

Figure 8. Formation of a translocation chromosome by breakage and rejoining of the major parts of two chromosomes into a single "translocation" chromosome (with the loss of the tiny broken pieces). When the fertilized egg receives this 14/21 translocation chromosome plus the usual two 21 chromosomes, the result will be a baby with translocation 21 trisomy Down's syndrome. When the fertilized egg receives the 14/21 translocation chromosome plus one 21 chromosome, the result will be a normal balanced translocation carrier, who will have a significant risk of having a child with Down's syndrome.

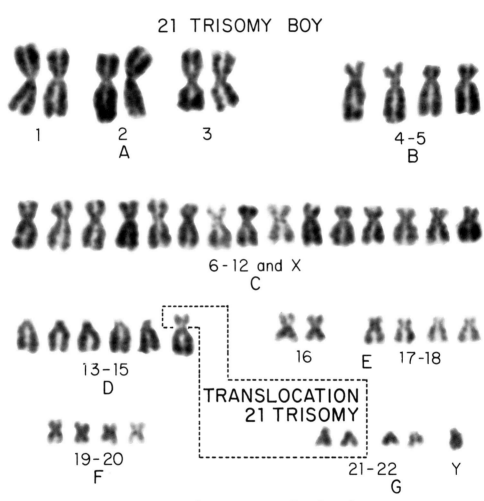

Figure 9.   Chromosomes of a child with translocation 21 trisomy Down's syndrome. There are 46 chromosomes, and the extra 21 chromosome long arm is attached to one of the D group chromosomes.

be 46. One chromosome will appear to have an extra piece attached to it, which is a large part of the extra 21 chromosome. As we have said, in the event of a translocation, it is important to examine the chromosomes of both parents to be sure that neither of them is a balanced carrier of the translocation.

WHO SHOULD HAVE A CHROMOSOME STUDY? When a child is born who has the physical appearance of Down's syndrome, the doctor must decide whether a chromosome study should be done. If there is any doubt about the diagnosis, or if he thinks the baby may have trisomy 21/normal mosaicism, a chromosome check is a wise idea. However, the physical features of a baby with Down's syndrome are usually sufficiently characteristic to permit the doctor to make a decision without a chromosome study. A chromosome study is advisable to exclude the possibility of a translocation if the mother is under 30 and plans to have more children. Translocations are unusual in Down's syndrome babies of older mothers, and a chromosome study is usually not necessary for babies born to women over 30 or 35, when the physical diagnosis is certain.

General Risk and Recurrence Risk for Down's Syndrome

What are the general chances of a family having a child with Down's syndrome, and after one, of having a second? It is important to remember that faults in chromosome distribution are not rare. At least 4 per cent of pregnancies begin with an unbalanced chromosome set in the beginning cell. Most of these pregnancies end in miscarriage shortly afterward because most genetic imbalances do not allow for the continued development of the growing embryo. In fact, one-fourth of all embryos lost by spontaneous miscarriage have an altered number of chromosomes. The presence of three number 21 chromosomes in the early cells does not have as severe an effect on development as the presence in triplicate of most of the other chromosomes.

The general risk of Down's syndrome must always be considered in relation to maternal age. As a woman reaches the latter years of her reproductive life, the likelihood of a fault in chromosome distribution increases progressively. Thus, after the age of 30 the likelihood of Down's syndrome approximately doubles for each successive 5-year period, as shown in Figure 10. At present, older maternal age is the only clear-cut human factor known to increase the likelihood of faulty chromosome distribution and Down's syndrome.

Figure 11 sets forth the recurrence risks for this disorder after a mother has had one child with Down's syndrome.

Prebirth Detection of Down's Syndrome

For those parents who have a relatively high risk of having a child with Down's syndrome, it is possible to do a chromosome study early in a pregnancy to determine whether the developing fetus has a chromosomal abnormality or not. The fetal cells are obtained from the amniotic fluid,

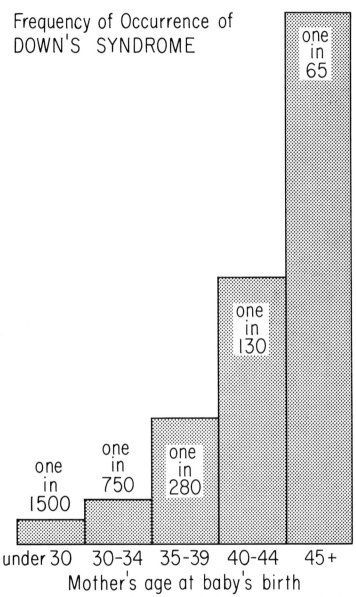

Frequency of Occurrence of
DOWN'S SYNDROME

one in 65

one in 130

one in 280

one in 750

one in 1500

under 30   30-34   35-39   40-44   45+
Mother's age at baby's birth

Figure 10. The general risk of having a child with Down's syndrome is related to the mother's age, and the risk increases progressively in women beyond 30 to 35 years of age. The approximate risks are given with each column. (Adapted from Mikkelsen, M., and Stene, J.: *Human Heredity* 20:457, 1970.)

DOWN'S SYNDROME RECURRENCE POSSIBILITY

CHROMOSOMES STUDIED

CHILD	PARENTS	RECURRENCE PROBABILITY
Full 21 trisomy	Chromosome studies rarely indicated	Mother under 30*–about 1% Over 30*– normal risk for age
Translocation 21 trisomy	Normal (most common)	Normal risk for age
	Mother balanced translocation carrier	10% or higher**
	Father balanced translocation carrier	2% or higher**

CHROMOSOMES NOT STUDIED

Mother under 30*	1% – 2%
Mother over 30*	Normal risk for age

*Mother's age at birth of Down's Syndrome child

**This is the most common type of translocation. Other types have other recurrence probability %'s.

Figure 11. Approximate risks of recurrence of Down's syndrome in subsequent children of parents who have had one affected child.

which surrounds the fetus. A small amount of the fluid is withdrawn by insertion of a needle through the pregnant woman's lower abdominal wall and uterus and into the fetal amniotic fluid space. This procedure, called amniocentesis, usually cannot be done before the thirteenth or fourteenth week of the pregnancy. Chromosome studies on the cultured cells, if successful, will usually yield a result within two to three weeks. The parents can then decide whether they wish the pregnancy to be terminated or not. This procedure is currently being performed in some of the larger medical centers.

Ideally, it would be worthwhile to perform amniocentesis and chromosome studies in all pregnancies and thereby prevent the birth of babies with Down's syndrome or other chromosomal abnormalities, which occur in one in 200 babies born. However, at the present time the risk of amniocentesis to a normal fetus has not been sufficiently clarified to fully warrant this as a routine procedure. The risk to the normal fetus appears to be small, the mortality rate being less than one in 200 fetuses studied, and hence the procedure definitely merits consideration in the following situations, in decreasing order of relative risk for occurrence of Down's syndrome and, therefore, decreasing order of consideration for amniocentesis:

1. The pregnant woman is a balanced 21 chromosome translocation carrier.

2. The father-to-be is a balanced 21 chromosome translocation carrier.

3. The couple has had more than one child with 21 trisomy Down's syndrome.

4. The prospective mother is in the older age group (especially those over 40 years of age).

5. The woman has had one full 21 trisomy Down's syndrome child.

Summary

1. The occurrence of Down's syndrome is due to a genetic imbalance, caused by the presence of an extra set of 21 chromosome genes. This genetic imbalance is most commonly due to a fault in chromosome distribution which occurs in the development of egg or the sperm or in the first division of the fertilized egg. This does not mean that any abnormal gene is present, and no event during the pregnancy can possibly be the cause of Down's syndrome.

2. The fault in chromosome distribution at cell division that gives rise to trisomy 21 is more likely to occur with older maternal age. The mother of a child with full trisomy 21 has about a 1 per cent risk of having another child with Down's syndrome if she is under the age of 30. If she is over 30 years the risk is about the same as that for any woman of the same age.

3. In a small minority of instances, the cause of Down's syndrome is translocation 21 trisomy. In this situation, the third number 21 chromosome is attached to another chromosome. In most cases this is a fresh occurrence, and for the chromosomally normal parents there is a very small risk (less than 1 per cent) that any future child will have Down's syn-

drome. However, in about one-third of these 21 trisomy translocation cases, one physically and mentally normal parent is found to be a balanced translocation carrier with a relatively high risk for recurrence.

4. Physical examination of a child with Down's syndrome does not distinguish between the full 21 trisomy and the translocation 21 trisomy type. This distinction can be made only by a chromosome study. It may be worthwhile for a child with Down's syndrome born to a young mother to have a chromosome check, but it usually is an unnecessary procedure for the Down's syndrome child of an older mother.

5. For those parents who have a relatively high recurrence risk for Down's syndrome, future pregnancies can be monitored by chromosome studies on fetal amniotic cells, with early termination of the pregnancy when the fetus is destined to have Down's syndrome.

REFERENCES

Carter, C. O., and Evans, K. A.: Risk of parents who have had one child with Down's syndrome (mongolism) having another child similarly affected. *Lancet* 2:785–788, 1961.

Collmann, R. D., and Stoller, A.: A survey of mongoloid births in Victoria Australia, 1942–1957. *American Journal of Public Health* 52:813–829, 1962.

Lilienfeld, A. M., and Benesch, C. H.: *Epidemiology of Mongolism.* The Johns Hopkins Press, Baltimore, 1969.

Mikkelsen, M., and Stene, J.: Genetic counselling in Down's syndrome. *Human Heredity* 20:457–464, 1970.

Penrose, L. S., and Smith, G. F.: *Down's Anomaly.* Little, Brown and Company, Boston, 1966.

Richards, B. W., Stewart, A., Sylverster, P. E., and Jasiewicz, V.: Cytogenetic survey of 225 patients diagnosed clinically as mongols. *Journal of Mental Deficiency* 9:245–259, 1965.

Sigler, A. T., Lilienfeld, A. M., Cohen, B. H., and Westlake, J. E.: Parental age in Down's syndrome (mongolism). *Journal of Pediatrics* 67:631–642, 1967.

Wright, S. W., Day, R. W., and Weinhouse, R.: The frequency of trisomy and translocation in Down's syndrome. *Journal of Pediatrics* 70:420–424, 1970.

2

What is a Child with Down's Syndrome Like? The Physical, Mental, and Social Characteristics of Down's Syndrome

What will a child with Down's syndrome be like as he grows up? What will he look like? Will he have serious health problems? What will his level of intelligence be, and how much can we teach him? Will he have a nice personality and get along well with people? Questions like these are almost always asked by parents of a baby with Down's syndrome. It is important for them to understand what he is most apt to be like as a baby, as a child, and as an adult before they make many of the decisions concerning his future.

Of course, truly accurate predictions can never be made about any given child; each has his own individuality from birth, and the effects of time and events will mold and shape his personality as well. In this chapter we try, however, to suggest what is usual for most children with Down's syndrome.

All the features that make up Down's syndrome occur because of the genetic imbalance. Trisomy 21, the presence of an extra 21 chromosome, is the primary cause of the child's altered pattern of physical and mental development. Children with Down's syndrome have some similarities to children with other types of mental deficiency or physical defect, but it is usually best not to compare them too closely. Trisomy 21 produces a particular blending of physical and mental characteristics, and of personality and behavior, that is unique to Down's syndrome children and often makes them stand out as a group, so that they are identifiable in a classroom or institution.

But just as these children have a certain uniqueness within the total spectrum of mentally deficient children, so each child with Down's syndrome has his own particular individuality. He has a personality and set of capabilities that are like those of no other person. The genetic imbalance causing Down's syndrome allows for considerable variability, which is reflected in each child's potential for mental and physical development. For example, one child may have an intelligence well below the average for Down's syndrome, while another, though mentally deficient, may seem relatively bright and alert. Some of these children may have more serious physical problems than the rest. So while this chapter presents the usual picture for Down's syndrome, it is important to remember that each child will vary to some degree from the common pattern.

There are three sections in the chapter. The first presents the features of growth, physical appearance, and health frequently seen in children with Down's syndrome. The second section deals with the development of the brain, the range of intelligence, social adjustability, and personality traits. In the last section, some of the serious physical problems that occur more frequently in Down's syndrome are discussed, as well as the most common causes of death in Down's syndrome babies.

I. The Most Common Physical Features and Health Problems of Down's Syndrome Children

The trisomy 21 that causes Down's syndrome affects many areas of physical development. The alterations it can produce vary greatly in their effect on growth and health; some are quite serious, while others hardly matter at all. The most serious effect is the alteration in development of the brain that occurs in every child with Down's syndrome. In less than half of the children, there is also a serious defect in development of the heart. The other serious alterations occur fairly infrequently, and most of them are discussed at the end of this section. Happily, many of the physical changes are relatively minor, and they do not affect the child's health or care in any major way. They are of use primarily as an aid in making a diagnosis of Down's syndrome. Almost all of these physical alterations have taken place before the child is born, in the early development of tissues and organs. Thus, immediately after birth an experienced doctor or nurse can usually recognize the features of Down's syndrome, even though the baby *may not* look unusual to the parent at birth, or even during infancy. All Down's syndrome children have similarities in physical appearance. Still, each one is an individual and has his own combination of physical and performance characteristics. For example, it is extremely unlikely that any Down's syndrome child will have *all* of the physical features mentioned here.

Figure 12 shows the hand of a child with Down's syndrome and Figures 13 to 18 show the appearance of affected persons of various ages.

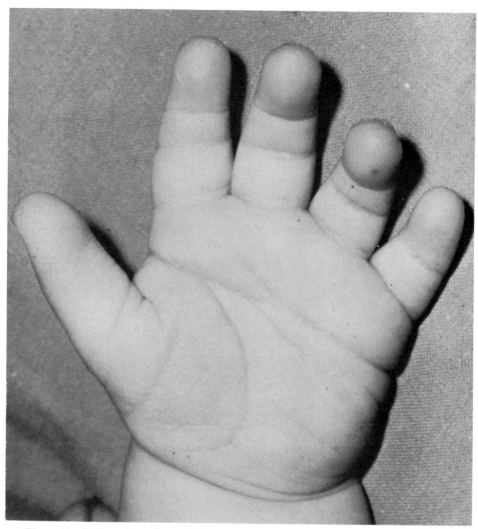

Figure 12. In Down's syndrome the hands and fingers tend to be shorter than usual, especially the little fingers. This may result in an altered crease pattern on the fifth finger and upper palm, as shown here, and the small finger may turn inward toward the others.

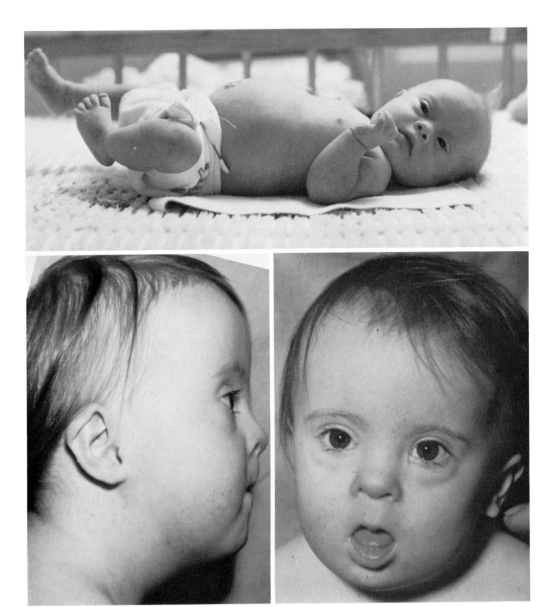

Figure 13. These two young infants with Down's syndrome demonstrate the individual variability in the typical features, which include a tendency toward a relatively low nasal bridge and small nose with flat facial contour, upslanting of the eye fissures with slight folds at the inner corner of the eye, fullness in lower eyelids, small ears, and a tendency to protrude the tongue. Many of these features change with age, as is shown in the ensuing photos. (Lower photographs from Smith, D. W.: *Recognizable Patterns of Human Malformation.* Philadelphia, W. B. Saunders Co., 1970.)

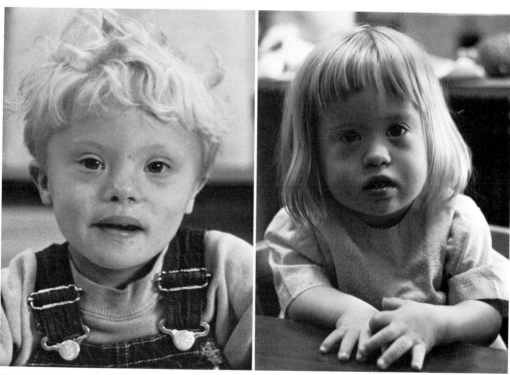

Figure 14.   Two year olds.

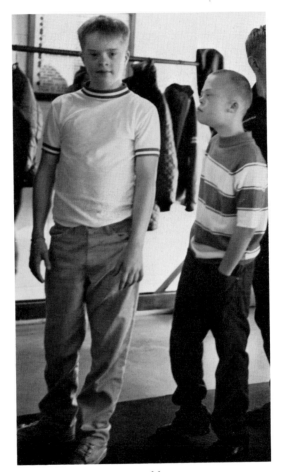

Figure 15.   Fourteen year olds.

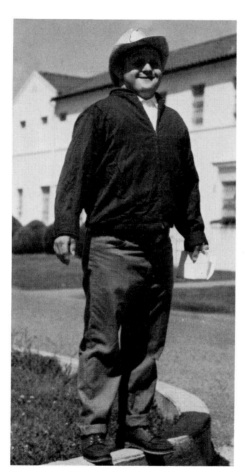

Figure 16.   Twenty-three year old.

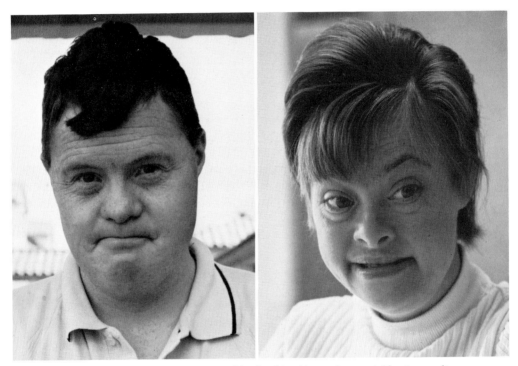

Figure 17.   Twenty-nine and thirty-one year old. The thin skin tends to wrinkle at an earlier age than usual.

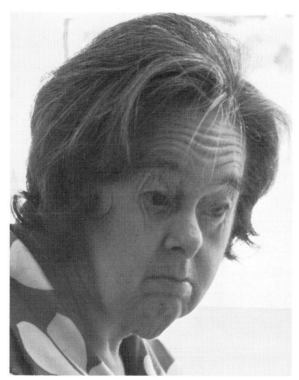

Figure 18.   Fifty-three year old.

Muscle Tone: Babies with Down's syndrome have less muscle tone (hypotonia) and therefore tend to be a bit "floppy" and loose-jointed. This improves with age and is seldom a problem.

Head: The back of the head (occiput) may appear less prominent than usual, and the head tends to be a bit smaller than average. The soft spots (fontanels) may be large and later in closing than usual.

Nose: The nose tends to be small, and the bridge of the nose somewhat low, so that, from a profile angle, the face appears relatively flat.

Eyes: The eyes tend to slant upward (slanting palpebral fissures). There may be small folds of skin at the inside corners of the eyes (inner canthal folds). These folds, which occasionally occur in normal babies, tend to become less prominent in later childhood. The outer portion of the iris of the eye may be speckled with lightly colored spots ("Brushfield spots"), especially noticeable in blue-eyed babies.

Ears: The ears are usually small, and sometimes prominent. The top rim of the ear (helix) is frequently folded over slightly. The ear lobes may be quite small.

Mouth: Although the tongue is of normal size, the mouth may be relatively small and the roof of the mouth a bit short; for this reason and because of generally poor muscle tone, the tongue of a baby with Down's syndrome may intermittently protrude. In older children with Down's syndrome a furrowed tongue sometimes develops. Their lips chap very easily out-of-doors.

Teeth: The teeth may be a bit small, and sometimes are abnormally shaped. They may come in late and occasionally are placed in an unusual position. Sometimes one or more teeth are missing. Children with Down's syndrome tend to have fewer cavities than other children. As they get older, they may have trouble with their gums, usually because the gums become inflamed or begin to recede. This may sometimes lead to loss of teeth in late childhood or early adulthood and is *not* necessarily due to poor oral hygiene.

Voice: The voice may have a slightly deep quality in early to late childhood. Onset of speech is generally late, and learning to talk articulately is generally difficult for Down's syndrome children. Some families have found that after their child has begun to talk, speech therapy can be of help if he is having difficulties in pronunciation and speech development.

Neck: The neck frequently appears a bit short. Babies with Down's syndrome may have loose folds of skin across the back of the neck which become less prominent with time.

Heart: In about 40 per cent of children with Down's syndrome a defect in the development of the heart is detected at birth or shortly afterward. In about half of these children the severity of the defect leads to an early death. The defects of heart development that may occur in Down's syndrome children are discussed in greater detail at the end of this chapter.

Hands: The hands often appear small, with relatively short fingers. There may be a single crease across the upper palm instead of the more usual two. The fifth finger may be somewhat short and may have only a single crease on it. The tip of this finger frequently turns inward toward the other fingers (clinodactyly).

Feet: There may be a small gap between the first and second toes, with a short crease running up between them on the sole of the foot.

Skin: The skin may have a mottled appearance and may become somewhat dry as the child grows older. Out-of-doors, his hands and face may chap easily.

Hair: The hair tends to be a bit sparse, fine, and straight.

Linear Growth: Children with Down's syndrome are, with rare exception, shorter than average and appear stocky in build because their arms and legs are a bit short in relation to the trunk. Birth length is usually within the normal range, and their growth up to about the age of 4 is only slightly behind the average for age. Around the age of 4 their rate of growth begins to fall below the normal range with each successive year. By age 15, a boy with Down's syndrome stands at the average height of an 8½-year-old. A 15-year-old girl with Down's syndrome stands at the average height of a 10-year-old. Like other children, they generally have a growth spurt during adolescence. The average final height of men with Down's syndrome is about 5 feet; the average height of women is 4 feet 7 inches. The graphs in Figures 19 and 20 show the average growth of children with Down's syndrome. With better nutrition and fewer serious infectious diseases, today's children with Down's syndrome are growing larger than in the past. Hence, do not be surprised if your Down's syndrome child exceeds these past expectations.

Weight Growth: Like length at birth, the birth weight of children with Down's syndrome tends to be low but is usually within the normal range. As they grow older, their weight, though low for age, corresponds with their shorter height. Mild to moderate obesity is not unusual in late childhood and adulthood. These children usually enjoy food, and parents may want to supervise the child's eating habits if obesity becomes a problem.

General Health in Childhood: About 20 to 40 per cent of babies with Down's syndrome do not survive the first few months or years. If a child with Down's syndrome does not have any of the more serious physical problems discussed at the end of this chapter, it is most likely that he will be healthy and will not present many difficulties in general care. He will be susceptible to the usual childhood illnesses and may have a few minor problems that other children do not have as often. For example, he may be more prone to minor infections, such as of the ear, eye, or respiratory tract, and may have more colds than his brothers and sisters. A runny nose can be a persistent problem even when other signs of a cold are absent. Later, it may help to encourage him to learn to use a handkerchief and blow his nose when necessary. A child with Down's syndrome requires normal dental care like other children, but may need special attention occasionally. While he probably will have a stocky build, it is not wise for him to become too overweight. He may have more accidents around the house and neighborhood because of his relatively poor coordination and judgment. Toilet training, bathing, and personal hygiene usually must be supervised to a later age than usual.

Adolescent and Sexual Development: Sexual development may be late in onset or incomplete or both. Males tend to produce less male hormone and may have a relatively small penis and less facial hair than usual. Females may have only mild to moderate breast development.

HEIGHT

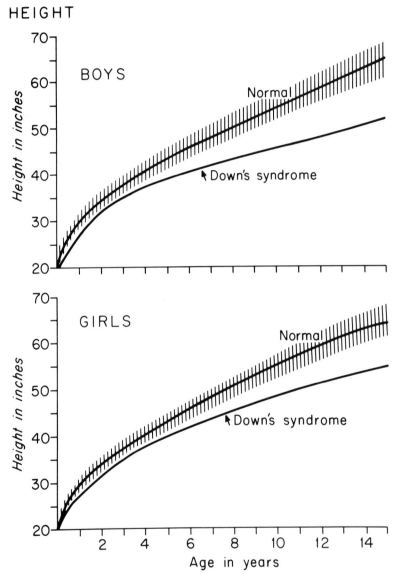

Figure 19. Average linear growth in Down's syndrome as contrasted to the normal growth rate. (Adapted from Thelander, H. E., and Pryor, H. B.: *Clinical Pediatrics* 5:493, 1966.)

WEIGHT

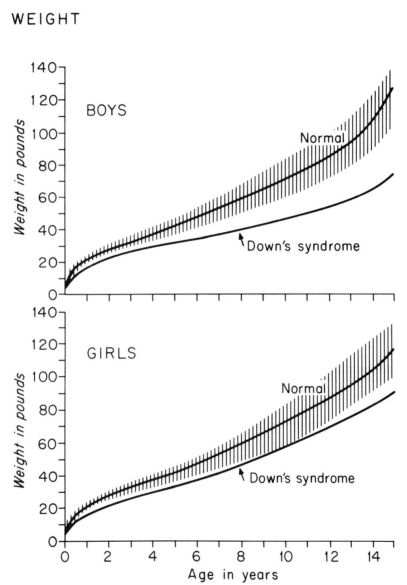

Figure 20.   Average weight growth in Down's syndrome as contrasted to the normal. (Adapted from Thelander, H. E., and Pryor, H. B.: *Clinical Pediatrics* 5:493, 1966.)

Menstruation usually begins at about the usual age and follows a normal course. Affected persons rarely marry, and their sexual drive is said to be diminished. Only a few Down's syndrome women have reproduced; about half their offspring have had Down's syndrome and half have been normal. This is to be expected, since the eggs of a woman with Down's syndrome would receive either two 21 chromosomes or one, and fertilization would yield 21 trisomy in the former case and a normal chromosome complement in the latter case. No man with Down's syndrome has ever been recorded as having fathered a child, and it is presumed that they are infertile.

Adulthood and Old Age: For those with Down's syndrome who survive the first few years, mortality rates are about the same as for normal persons until around age 40, when the rate begins to increase. Adults with Down's syndrome are susceptible to most of the illnesses and problems common to their environment and age group, but in some ways they seem to age more rapidly than normal. This aging process is most evident in the skin and in the mucous membranes of the mouth. For example, the skin of adults with Down's syndrome tends to become dry and somewhat coarse with time. In some the gums recede; this may result in premature loss of teeth. Respiratory infections, pneumonia, and lung disease can be a problem for some Down's syndrome adults and are one potential cause of death.

II. The Usual Mental and Social Characteristics of Down's Syndrome Children

The trisomy 21 that causes Down's syndrome always has an effect on the development and function of the brain. As you know, the brain controls many aspects of development, including muscle coordination, the five senses, intelligence, and many aspects of behavior. Considering the brain's complex and sensitive nature, it is not surprising that the genetic imbalance of a whole extra set of 21 chromosome genes produces alterations in the brain's development and potential. As a result, all children with Down's syndrome are mentally deficient to some degree.

The way in which trisomy 21 affects the brain is not clear. It is probably easiest to think of it as preventing the brain from developing to its usual size and complexity. The size of the brain can be judged roughly by measuring the circumference of a child's head. In Down's syndrome the head tends to be smaller than usual and increases in size at a somewhat slower rate than usual until about the age of 3, with relatively less growth after that age (see Figure 21). At the age of 15, both boys and girls with Down's syndrome most commonly have a head size, and thus a brain size, of a normal child of 2½ years. However, even though the head size is relatively small in proportion to the rest of the body, it is not a particularly striking feature, and people are usually unaware of it.

Like all children, the child with Down's syndrome has a pattern of mental development that parallels his pattern of brain growth. Every baby's brain at birth is incompletely developed. As the brain continues to develop rapidly in the first several years of life, the baby is able to do more and more. At a certain level of brain development, he is able to smile; later

HEAD CIRCUMFERENCE

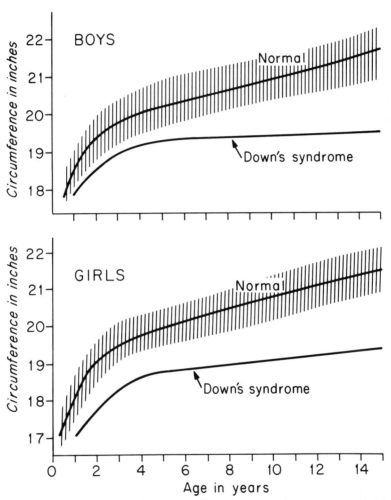

Figure 21.   Average head circumference growth in Down's syndrome as contrasted to the normal. (Adapted from Thelander, H. E., and Pryor, H. B.: *Clinical Pediatrics* 5:493, 1966.) Our own more recent data show larger head circumference in many children with Down's syndrome.

on its progress enables him to master sitting and walking; and still later he can talk, go without diapers, and dress himself. Children learn new skills throughout childhood as their advancing level of brain development allows their capabilities to expand. They advance from simple motor skills to more sophisticated activities like talking, reading, problem-solving, social adaptability, and independence.

In Down's syndrome children, however, the rate of mental development tends to be progressively slower as the brain's rate of development slows down. In their early years, they seem relatively alert and capable of performing some of the basic motor skills at a slower, but not too retarded pace. Later, however, it is difficult for them to learn more advanced skills. Their potential for intellectual development is set at a lower level. It is important that children with Down's syndrome be encouraged to develop all their abilities, to learn and achieve as much as their potential will allow. Most Down's syndrome children enjoy the stimulation and sense of accomplishment that learning brings. Education enables them to be productive to some degree in society, to make their own lives fuller, to place a smaller burden on those who care for them, and to have pride in their limited achievements. But it is important to remember that the extent of their achievements is determined largely by the development of the brain, which cannot be forced beyond its limits. As of the present, we know of no physician, educator, or psychologist who has found any consistent and accepted method for advancing brain growth or substantially improving a child's inborn capacity for mental development. Every child with Down's syndrome is different, and the potential of each one is different. There is a wide variability in the degree of mental deficiency, from the rare child who is severely defective to the occasional one who may attain an adult I.Q. of 60 or above. But the majority of children with Down's syndrome fall within a certain range, and this section deals with the abilities and mental potential which are usual for most of them.

When a baby with Down's syndrome is born, the fact that he is going to be mentally deficient may not seem at all obvious to those around him. He may seem a bit floppy and loose-jointed and have somewhat poor muscle tone. He probably will have no serious difficulty in feeding, although his suck may be a little weak. In most cases, the mother who wishes to breast-feed her baby can do so without much trouble. A baby with Down's syndrome generally seems fairly perky and alert, and will soon try to hold up his head and then roll over. He gurgles and develops a smile at about the same time other babies do. The ability to sit and walk alone usually comes at a later age than usual. Figure 22 gives a rough comparison of when normal children and those with Down's syndrome who are raised at home develop some of the early skills. It is noteworthy that the range of variability for Down's syndrome children is much greater than for normal children.

The environment in which the Down's syndrome child is raised does appear to make some difference in his rate of early progress in performance. In general, children with Down's syndrome raised at home with the normal amount of stimulation advance more quickly than those who spend their early years in an institution for the mentally deficient. For example, in a recent study, the ages at which children with Down's syndrome raised at home first walked were compared with those of children

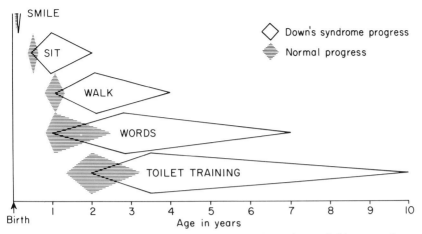

Figure 22. Early development performance of Down's syndrome children raised at home compared to that of normal children. The widest point in each diamond represents the average age for performance, and the spread of the diamonds represents the range.

who were raised in an institution. Forty-four per cent of children at home walked by age 2, 78 per cent by age 3, and 95 per cent by age 5. Of those in institutions, none walked by age 2, 6 per cent walked by age 3, and 84 per cent walked by age 5. As these figures show, Down's syndrome children raised at home learn to walk much earlier than those in institutions, but by the age of 5 most of those in institutions also are walking. It appears, then, that most children with Down's syndrome have the capability to walk. When they are able to actually do so seems largely dependent on their environment and the encouragement they receive.

In some institutions it is now possible to give each child more individualized attention, which helps speed up some aspects of their early development. Another study of development of Down's syndrome children compared those raised at home with those raised in an institutional setting that was "enriched" with more staff members, pleasant surroundings, and other Down's syndrome children of similar ages nearby. Both groups of children learned to walk at about the same time, the average age being 27 months.

The ability to talk comes a great deal later for a child with Down's syndrome than the ability to walk. Speech involves much more than just being able to pronounce words. A child must first understand what the words mean, know what he wants to say, and comprehend what people say to him in response. This process requires more "thinking" than the relatively simpler motor skills he has probably already mastered. Whereas the normal child can generally say a few words by the age of 1 year, the child with Down's syndrome who is raised at home can usually do so only at 2 to 3 years. Again, the range is great; some may say words at a year, and others not until the age of 7 or 8. An institutionalized child may possibly learn a few words on his own at a later age, but it seems that stimulating a child with Down's syndrome to talk requires a much greater amount of personal contact than most institutions can provide. Even in the "enriched" institution in the study just mentioned, the children learned to talk less quickly than those raised at home. The "enriching" elements of the institution had less beneficial effect on learning to speak than on learning to walk. Apparently the time and effort a mother puts into encouraging her child to say his first words simply cannot be duplicated in an institution.

Living at home, a child with Down's syndrome can often accomplish a variety of small jobs with some encouragement and training. These activities usually are simple ones, requiring gross eye-to-hand coordination and lots of repetition and practice. A child with Down's syndrome generally can learn to do such things as dress and feed himself, play on a swing, swim, set the table, and rake leaves. In contrast, activities that require finer eye-to-hand coordination, speech, and the more "intellectual" skills are much harder for a child with Down's syndrome to accomplish. Even in his teens and beyond, tasks requiring independence and responsibility will be difficult for him. For example, an average teen-ager with Down's syndrome probably cannot read and write very well, or safely drive a car, or look after a younger child. These children never seem to gain the maturity and judgment that other children develop with age and experience.

A teen-ager or adult with Down's syndrome usually has the intellectual capabilities of a young child. Although in his early years he may appear relatively bright and alert, his rate of progress gradually slows down and levels off, as the chart in Figure 23 indicates. If a young child with Down's syndrome is given an I.Q. test before the age of 4 or 5 years, his parents may find themselves encouraged by the score. But it is most unlikely that the child will be able to maintain his early rate of performance, and his I.Q. scores will usually drop progressively as time goes by. The average I.Q. scores of older children and adults with Down's syndrome

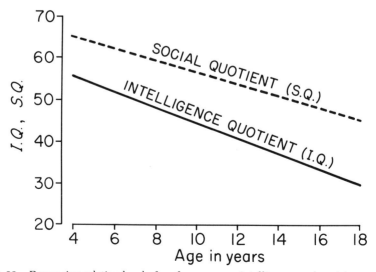

Figure 23. Decreasing relative level of performance on intelligence and social performance testing with age in Down's syndrome, as compared to normal. (Adapted from Cornwell, A. C., and Birth, H. G.: *American Journal of Mental Deficiency* 74:341, 1969.)

range between 25 and 50. This fall in I.Q. scores does not mean that Down's syndrome children deteriorate with age, but only that they do not maintain their early pace and that they reach their final level of intellectual development at an earlier age than normal persons do.

Actual intelligence scores are somewhat misleading in the assessment of the capabilities of a Down's syndrome child or adult. Even though his mental age may compare most closely with that of a child of 4 to 6 years old, the adult with Down's syndrome can be taught some things that a normal child might have difficulty learning. For example, some families who live in rural areas have been able to teach their Down's syndrome children to run a tractor; other families have found these children can learn to do housework, run a factory machine, or do simple carpentry.

Perhaps more important, the social development of Down's syndrome children is often 2 or 3 years more advanced than their level of mental development (see Figure 23). Consequently, they may appear to be more intelligent than they really are, and can deal more easily with their environment and the people they live with than their mental abilities might suggest. They can often fit comfortably into a family group, provided the family is comfortable around them. In general, they are cheerful, friendly, outgoing, and active (even boisterous at times), though many have a stubborn streak. They enjoy people and have a flair for mimicry; they like to imitate people and do things as others do them. This makes it possible to teach them manners and to try to behave as their brothers and sisters do. They like to eat dinner with the rest of the family, go on outings, and attend a special school or day care center with other children. Langdon Down, the physician who first described the features of Down's syndrome in 1866, gave the following description of the personalities of several Down's syndrome children he had under his care.

> Several patients ... have been wont to convert their pillowslips into surplices and to imitate, in tone and gesture, the clergyman chaplain they have recently heard. . . . I have known a ventriloquist to be convulsed with laughter between the first and second parts of his entertainment on seeing a patient mount the platform, and hearing him imitate the performance with which the audience had been entertained. They have a strong sense of the ridiculous; this is indicated by their humourous remarks and the laughter with which they hail accidental falls, even of those to whom they are most attached. Another feature is their great obstinacy—they can only be guided by consummate tact. No amount of coercion will induce them to do that which they have made up their minds not to do. . . They are always amiable both to their companions and to animals. They are not passionate nor strongly affectionate.

Children with Down's syndrome usually take great pleasure in their surroundings, their families, their toys, their playmates. Happiness comes easily, and throughout life they usually maintain a childlike good humor. They are not burdened with the grown-up cares that come to most people with adolescence and adulthood. They never feel the pressures of applying to college, supporting and raising a family, or working hard for job promotions, because they never develop that degree of responsibility and maturity. Life is simpler and less complex. The emotions that others feel seem to be less intense for them. They are sometimes sad, happy, angry, or irritable, like everyone else, but their moods are generally not so profound and they blow away more quickly. Sexual and aggressive passions also are much more muted. An adolescent boy with Down's syndrome will probably never cause any problem in the neighborhood with young girls. As we mentioned earlier, the men are believed to be infertile.

Stubbornness is perhaps the most unpleasant personality trait of persons with Down's syndrome. They can sometimes be extremely obstinate and determined to have their own way. This calls for perseverance and firmness on the part of parents; it is important to establish discipline early, and to make clear who is boss.

Sometimes in children who are mentally deficient certain areas of mental development and function are more acute than others. Occasionally these areas are even more strongly developed than in normal people. Most children with Down's syndrome have an increased sensitivity to music. They love rhythm and dance, and often are good at playing simple musical instruments, percussion and rhythm instruments especially. Listening to music, singing, dancing, or playing an instrument brings them great pleasure.

A child with Down's syndrome, though slow, is still very responsive to his environment, to those around him, and to the affection and encouragement he receives from others. Most families, including foster families, provide a child with a great deal of attention, and they enjoy encouraging him to take his first steps or say his first words. Most institutions cannot provide this kind of constant teaching and stimulation, and on the average, the I.Q. scores of Down's syndrome children raised in institutions are 10 or 15 points lower than those of children who live in a home setting. The early years are the most important ones for a Down's syndrome child because it is then that his development proceeds at its greatest pace. A child who spends his first 3 or 4 years at home usually can accomplish much more than a child who is reared in an institution from birth. If the child from home is then placed in an institution, he still usually performs better than those children raised there, but his rate of progress drops off more rapidly than if he had remained at home. Today many institutions understand the importance of early education and training in fostering a child's abilities to perform useful skills, and many now provide children with the opportunity to learn skills and simple trades that they can be proud of and that can even be useful to the local community. Some mental retardation centers have established programs in which brighter Down's syndrome teen-agers and adults can live together under supervision in the community, maintaining limited jobs and partially supporting themselves.

It is nice to know that children with Down's syndrome do not necessarily lose their good humor when they live in an institution with pleasant surroundings. They tend to enjoy life wherever they find it and they particularly like the company of other Down's syndrome children. They seek each other out and can be quite clannish. Visitors to an institution, seeing Down's syndrome children together, often have the same pleasant reaction as the doctor who, upon leaving, remarked with surprise, "How happy they all are!"

In sum, the inborn potential for growth and development of a child with Down's syndrome, while much more limited than that of a normal child, does allow him to acquire some skills that make life livable and pleasant. He usually can master walking, a limited amount of speech, self-care, and some of the more intellectual skills. But perhaps more important, a child with Down's syndrome generally is born with a cheerful and loving nature, which can bring happiness to others as well as himself.

III. Serious Physical Problems Associated with Down's Syndrome

The first section of this chapter presented the physical features that children with Down's syndrome have in common. In this section some of the more serious physical problems associated with Down's syndrome are discussed. While they are not the common features, they occur much more frequently in Down's syndrome children than in normal children. One-third to one-half of all babies born with Down's syndrome have one of these more serious problems. The trisomy 21 that causes Down's syndrome is responsible for all the alterations in development, the relatively minor ones as well as those of a more serious nature. The effects of the genetic imbalance may be much more severe in one child than in another. There is no correlation between the number of physical problems present in a Down's syndrome child and his degree of mental deficiency, and the fact that he has a physical defect does not reflect in any way on his family or on the mother's pregnancy. The presence of a serious physical defect in a Down's syndrome child does not increase the risk of any future child without Down's syndrome having the same defect.

Susceptibility to Infection: Children with Down's syndrome, especially young infants, often have minor defects in their body's defense mechanism against infectious diseases. They are more likely to have infections in the lungs (pneumonia), or in the intestine (gastroenteritis). In the past, these types of infection, particularly pneumonia, were the major causes of death in babies with Down's syndrome. Today, pneumonia and gastroenteritis are much less common in all children, including those with Down's syndrome. Modern antibiotic drugs have greatly reduced the number of deaths from pneumonia, and Down's syndrome children seem to respond to treatment about as well as normal children. This may not be true when there is also a serious problem in the development of the heart.

Heart Problems: In about 30 to 40 per cent of all Down's syndrome babies development of the heart is incomplete. Most commonly, an opening has been left between the two sides of the heart where a partition should normally have formed. If the opening is very large, the function of the heart may be poor, and the baby is often lethargic and inactive. A doctor can usually determine soon after birth whether or not there is a serious heart defect. A minor defect may disappear with time, or have no effects on the child's later growth, health, or activity. If the baby's heart is normally formed, there is no concern about heart problems during childhood.

Problems in the Intestinal Tract: About 4 per cent of Down's syndrome babies are born with incomplete development of the intestine. There are several areas in which the intestinal tract can fail to develop properly. There can be blockage in the tube leading to the stomach (esophagus), or, more commonly, blockage just beyond the stomach in the duodenum (2.4 per cent of Down's syndrome babies). Also, the lower part of the large intestine can be in an abnormal position, or the last part of the large bowel may be unable to function (Hirschsprung's disease), or the anal opening may be missing. Blockage above the stomach usually causes a baby to vomit at the first feedings. Blockage below the stomach causes the baby's stomach (abdomen) to enlarge, and vomiting begins during the first day or two. Because serious alterations in the development of the intestinal tract usually cause some kind of difficulty in a baby's normal feeding or bowel movements, these are generally the first clues that something may be wrong. They appear in the first days or, at most, weeks after the child's birth. If no problem in the development of the intestine becomes obvious during the first several months, there need be little concern that any will appear later.

About one in every eight babies with Down's syndrome has a small protrusion of the navel (umbilical hernia), which is not a serious problem.

Eye Problems: Eye problems are relatively common and vary in severity. Often the eyes of Down's syndrome babies tend to cross because the proper coordination between them is slow in developing fully. This crossing, called strabismus, generally improves with age. If it does not by the time the child is 1 to 2 years old, surgery may be indicated to correct it. Strabismus does not necessarily interfere with the child's vision.

More common eye problems are simple errors in refraction, such as nearsightedness, which glasses can usually remedy. A cloudiness in the lens of the eye (cataract) may develop at a later age and may rarely be present at birth.

Other Problems: Leukemia, an uncontrolled growth of white blood cells that is generally fatal, occurs in about 1 per cent of Down's syndrome children. Usually the disease is of the acute type and develops in the first 2 or 3 years, the risk thereafter being low. Babies with leukemia do not survive longer than a few months without treatment; with treatment they may live another year or two.

One-half per cent of Down's syndrome children have a cleft lip or cleft palate. Another 1 per cent have a foot placed in an abnormal position (clubfoot) which requires temporary wearing of a cast for improvement.

About 15 per cent of Down's syndrome children have some kind of serious behavioral problem. It is always difficult to determine the exact cause of these problems, especially in a mentally deficient child. Some of them may be due to an unloving or insecure home situation, others to the stress of coping with the pressures of life in a "normal" world. Many may be due to an unusual variation in the child's brain development which affects his behavior; in these cases, the parents are not responsible in any way for the problem.

There are several other physical problems that are seen more frequently in children with Down's syndrome than in normal children, but they occur in less than one-half per cent of Down's syndrome children and need not be mentioned here.

THE MORTALITY RATE IN DOWN'S SYNDROME BABIES. In the past, a great many babies with Down's syndrome died in the first 2 years of life. Today the majority of them survive these early years. The decrease in the mortality rate is due to a general falloff in the occurrence of serious infectious disease among infants, and to the modern use of antibiotics in fighting certain types of pneumonia. Even in the recent past, however, the mortality rate has been relatively high. For example, from 1948 to 1957, the mortality of children with Down's syndrome in Victoria, Australia, was close to 50 per cent, the deaths occurring predominantly during early infancy. Our own recent experience indicates a lower mortality, about 20 to 30 per cent. The Australian study showed the mortality of affected persons from 5 to 40 years of age to be 4 to 7 per cent higher than normal, not a significant difference. After age 40, the mortality rate increased more rapidly, so that after 50 years it was 30 per cent above usual. It seems that adults with Down's syndrome age more rapidly than normal persons.

Today, defects in development of the heart are the major cause of death in young children with Down's syndrome. They account for two-thirds of deaths that occur during the first year of life. Other causes for early death are intestinal blockage, infection in the lung (pneumonia), and infection in the intestine (gastroenteritis). All of these serious problems that may cause death in a child with Down's syndrome occur because of the child's genetic imbalance. The trisomy 21 is the fundamental cause of all the alterations in development and function seen in Down's syndrome, and consequently is responsible for all the deaths in Down's syndrome children resulting from these alterations.

It is always difficult for parents to know what to do when they learn that their baby with Down's syndrome has a serious physical problem that threatens his life. There are three important things for them to understand before they make any decisions. First, parents should know what Down's syndrome is and how it will affect the life of the child. Second, they should have a good understanding of the seriousness of their child's physical problem and of the ways in which it will alter the child's life and function. Third, parents should know what options are open to them for treatment of their child's physical handicap, and how thorough and effective these methods are. As parents, they have the right to decide whether or not a potentially lifesaving or life-prolonging measure should be undertaken. For example, if the Down's syndrome baby is born with blockage in the intestinal tract that can be helped only by major surgery, the parents have the prerogative to either reject or request the surgery. Only the baby's parents or guardian can authorize surgery. Sometimes it is difficult to know ahead of time how successful surgery will be for a Down's syndrome infant, especially if the heart is involved. Some problems in heart development can be helped only by major open-heart surgery; sometimes the defect is extremely difficult to repair and surgery itself may threaten the baby's life, and sometimes the heart cannot be completely repaired. Also, there is at present no permanent cure for the 1 per cent of Down's syndrome children who have leukemia, but there is medication that can lead to temporary prolongation of life, and the parents should be allowed to determine whether such therapy should be utilized or not.

Parents should be open and frank in discussing their Down's syndrome child's problems with the doctor. Most doctors are sympathetic and understanding of parents' wishes, and it is important to speak honestly with him about the child and his care.

REFERENCES

Common Physical Features

Cohen, M. M., Sr., and Cohen, M. M., Jr.: The oral manifestations of trisomy G_1 (Down's syndrome). *Birth Defects: Original Article Series* 7:241–251, 1971.

Gustavson, K.-H.: *Down's Syndrome, a Clinical and Cytogenetical Investigation.* Almqvist & Wiksells, Uppsala, Sweden, 1964.

Penrose, L. S., and Smith, G. F.: *Down's Anomaly.* Little, Brown and Company, Boston, 1966.

Thelander, H. E., and Pryor, H. B.: Abnormal patterns of growth and development in mongolism. An anthropometric study. *Clinical Pediatrics* 5:493–501, 1966.

Mental and Social Characteristics

Centerwall, S. A., and Centerwall, W. R.: A study of children with mongolism reared in the home compared to those reared away from the home. *Pediatrics* 25:678–685, 1960.

Cornwell, A. C., and Birch, H. G.: Psychological and social development in home-reared children with Down's syndrome (mongolism). *American Journal of Mental Deficiency* 74:341–350, 1969.

Quaytman, W.: The psychological capacities of mongoloid children in a community clinic. *Quarterly Review of Pediatrics* 8:255–267, 1953.

Shipe, D., and Shotwell, A. M.: Effect of out-of-home care on mongoloid children: a continuation study. *American Journal of Mental Deficiency* 69:649–652, 1965.

Shotwell, A. M., and Shipe, D.: Effect of out-of-home care on the intellectual and social development of mongoloid children. *American Journal of Mental Deficiency* 68:693–699, 1964.

Stedman, O. J., and Eichorn, D. H.: A comparison of the growth and development of institutionalized and home-reared mongoloids during infancy and early childhood. *American Journal of Mental Deficiency* 69:391–401, 1964.

Serious Physical Problems

Carter, C. O.: A life-table for mongols with causes of death. *Journal of Mental Deficiency Research* 2:64–74, 1958.

Collmann, R. D., and Stoller, A.: A life-table for mongols in Victoria, Australia. *Journal of Mental Deficiency Research* 7:53–59, 1963.

Fabis, J., and Drolette, M.: Malformation and leukemia in children with Down's syndrome. *Pediatrics* 45:60–70, 1970.

Lillienfeld, A. M., and Benesch, C. H.: *Epidemiology of Mongolism.* The Johns Hopkins Press, Baltimore, 1969.

Penrose, L. S., and Smith, G. F.: *Down's Anomaly.* Little, Brown and Company, Boston, 1966.

Rowe, R. D., and Uchida, I. A.: Cardiac malformation in mongolism. *American Journal of Medicine* 31:726–735, 1961.

3

A Photo Album of Down's Syndrome Children

A VISIT WITH AMY AND HER PARENTS

Amy is only a month old and already is an active baby with a very appealing personality. She enjoys her surroundings and the fun of discovering what she can do with her arms and legs.

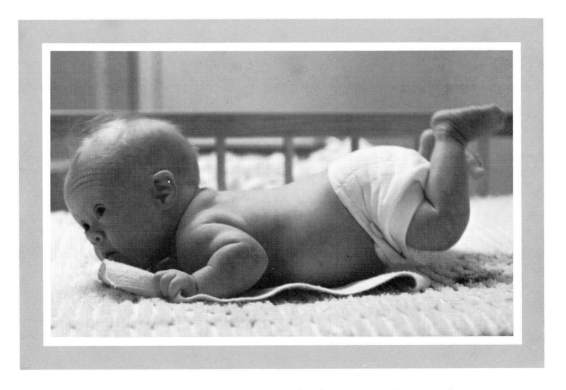

Amy demonstrates her flexibility by swinging her legs up into the air. Lifting her head and controlling its movements are harder for her.

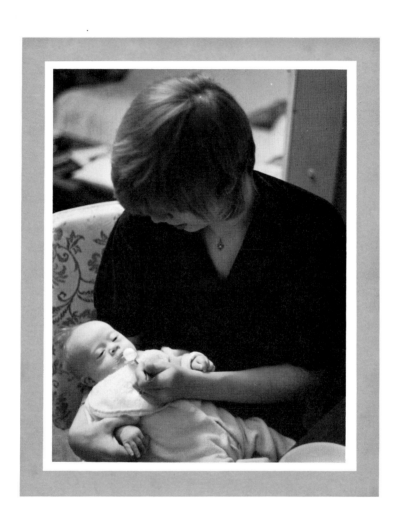

Amy samples cereal.

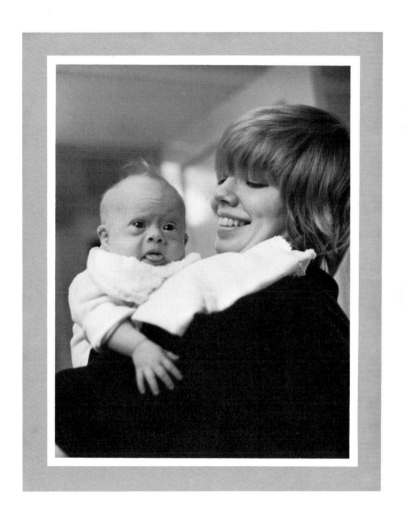

A good burp!

Amy's parents, Stephanie and Dick, are 19 years old and new to the task of caring for a baby. Below, Stephanie shows her husband the best way to hold the bottle for Amy's after-lunch milk. In a moment, everything is going well and Amy drinks her milk peacefully under the proud eyes of her parents. Afterward, Amy falls sound asleep on Dick's shoulder.

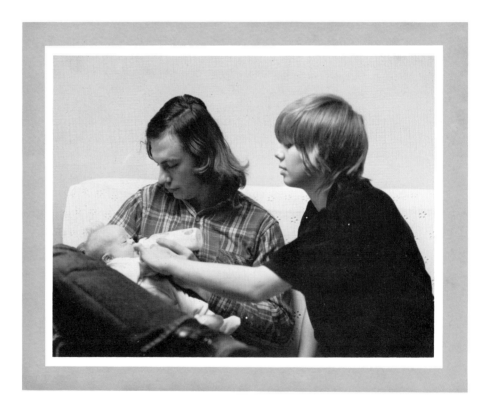

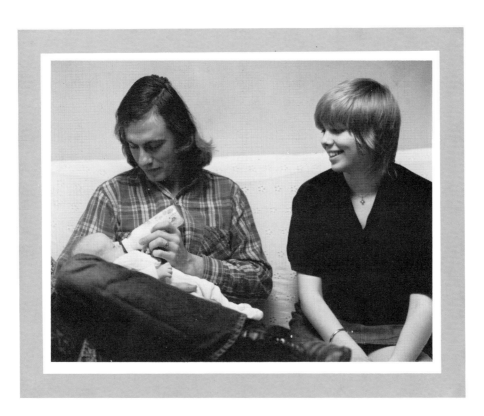

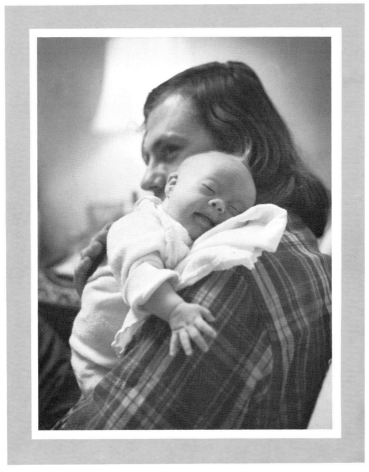

A VISIT WITH ALISON AND HER MOTHER

Alison is 14 months old and overflows with impishness and affection. She takes a real delight in life and is full of smiles for everyone. Below, Alison wakes up from her afternoon nap and plays pat-a-cake with her mother, who has come to wake her up. After a nice nap she is ready for her visitors, and grins happily for the camera. Her pretty face includes some of the typical features of Down's syndrome: the small nose, the folds in the corners of her eyes, her flat profile. Like many babies, Alison is intrigued by her own reflection in the mirror.

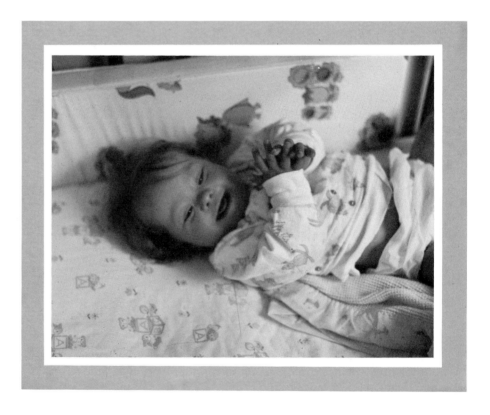

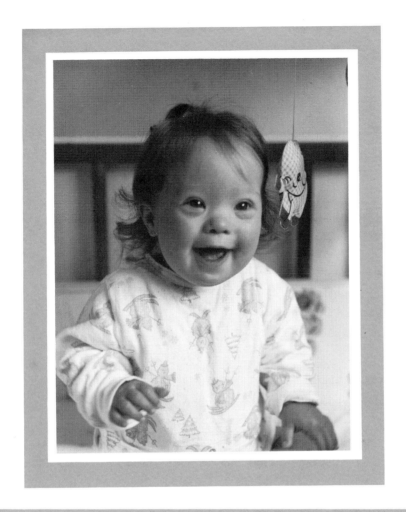

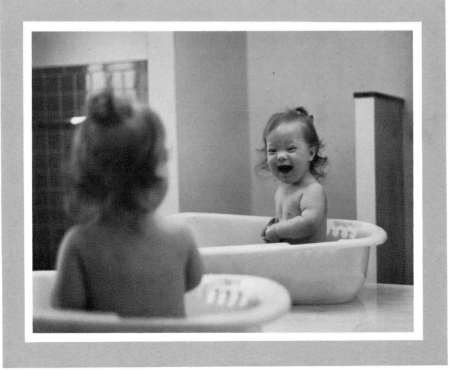

51

On a lovely spring day the place to be is outside in the sun. Alison and Joan, her mother, do some exercises and practice standing. Alison's development is slow, but on schedule for Down's syndrome. Joan spends a lot of time working with her, and they have just begun classes several mornings a week at a nearby school for the mentally deficient to help Alison develop motor skills. Her parents are eager to encourage Alison's development, especially in her early years when progress is usually most rapid for Down's syndrome children.

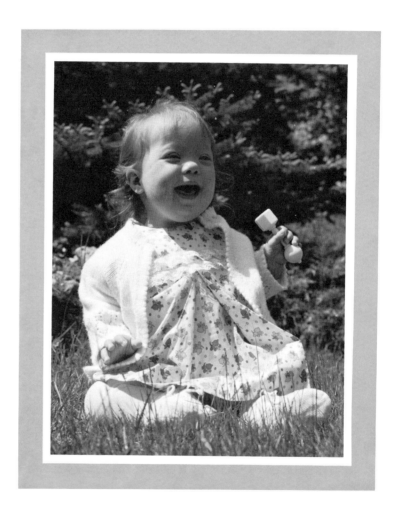

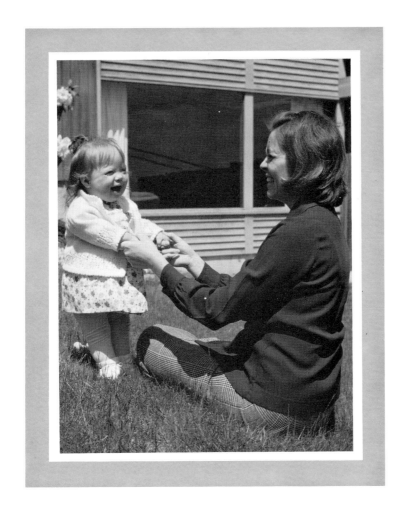

Alison at dinnertime is a kaleidoscope of smiles and tears, hungry looks, dirty face, and lots of mess.

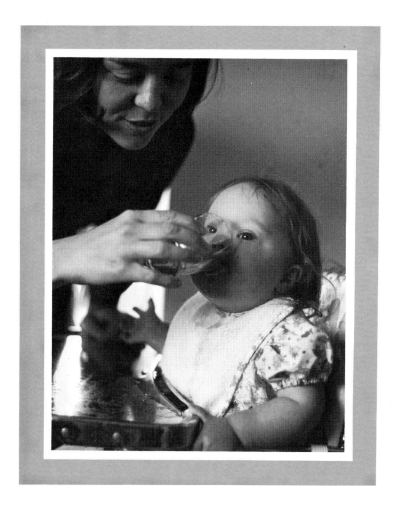

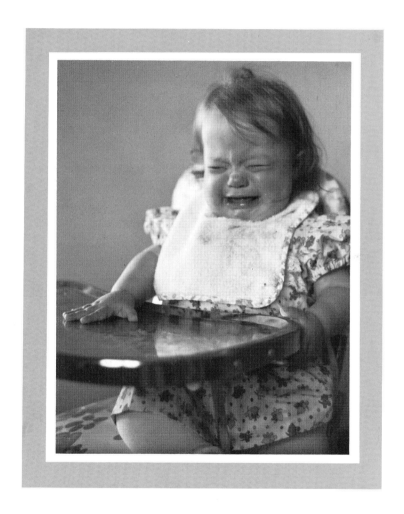

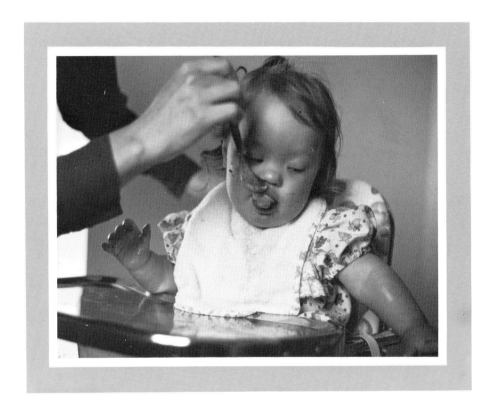

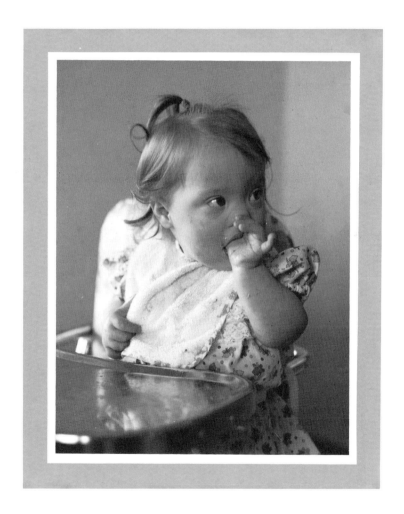

A VISIT TO THE PRE-SCHOOL FOR DOWN'S SYNDROME CHILDREN AT THE UNIVERSITY OF WASHINGTON

This experimental pre-school takes about a dozen children, who range in age from just under 2 to just over 3. There are five teachers and parent volunteers who work with the youngsters. Each child gets a lot of individual attention and one-to-one help. In each class there are opportunities to play with all kinds of toys: blocks, paint, clay, musical instruments. Interspersed throughout the class period are lessons in walking and other gross motor skills. Each child also receives a concentrated lesson in fine motor coordination.

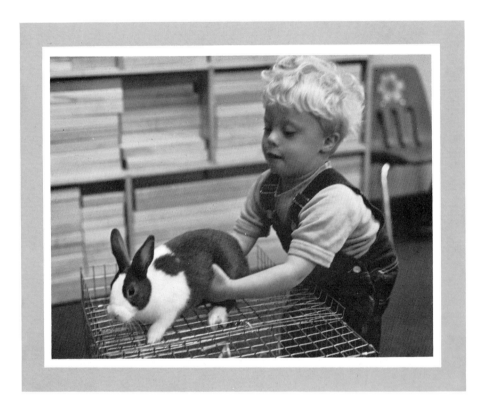

Dennis pays a visit to the rabbit who lives by the window.

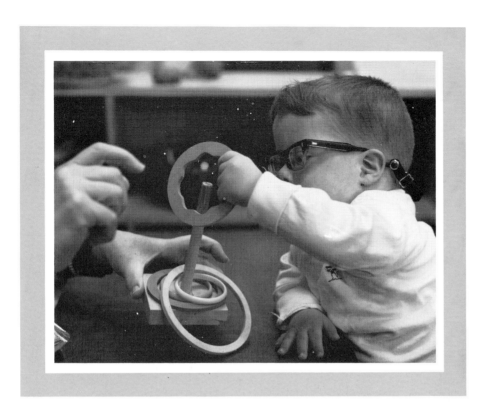

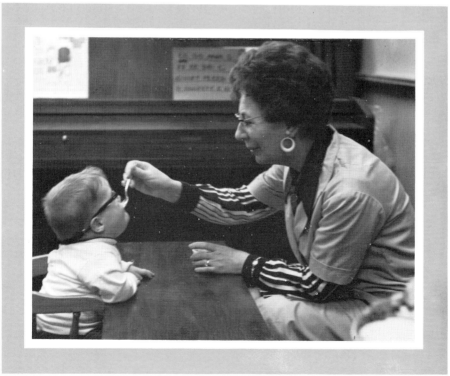

Jamie learns to drop a hoop . . . over the stick . . . and gets a taste of ice cream as a reward.

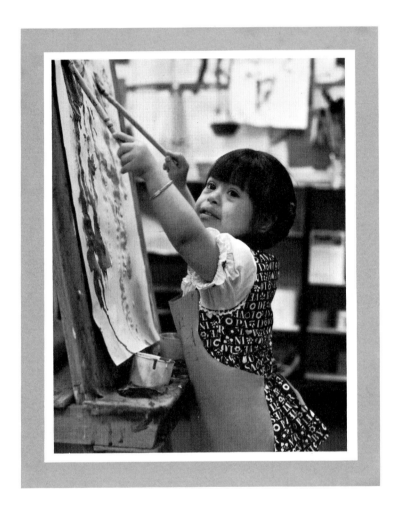

Lupita paints . . .

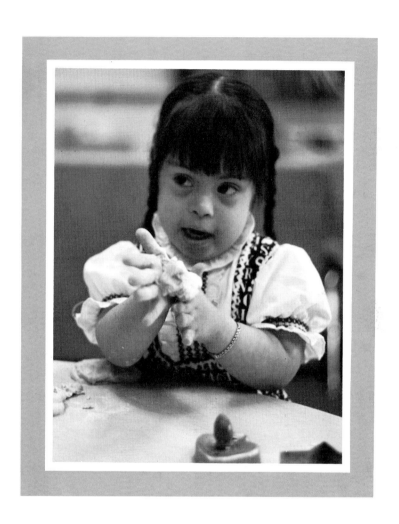

. . . and makes cookies.

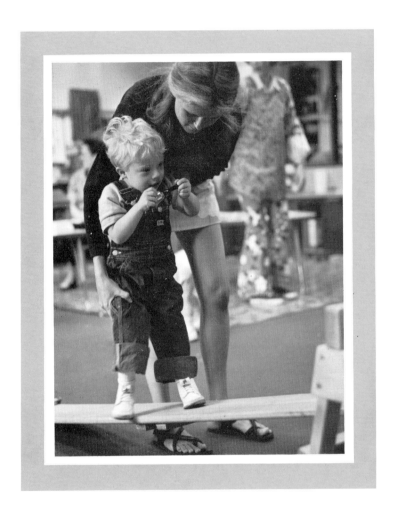

Dennis being helped to develop better balance.

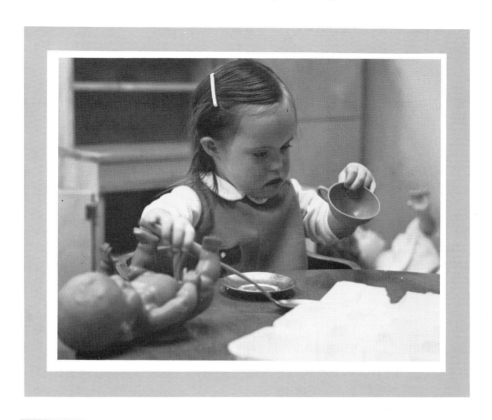

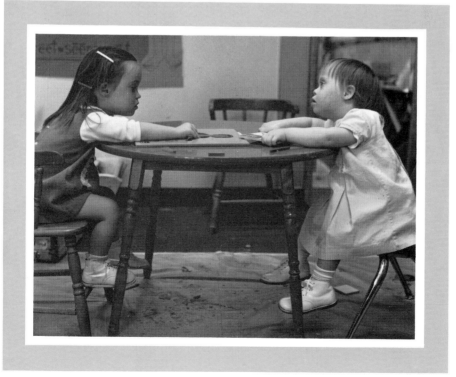

Time for work and time for contemplation.

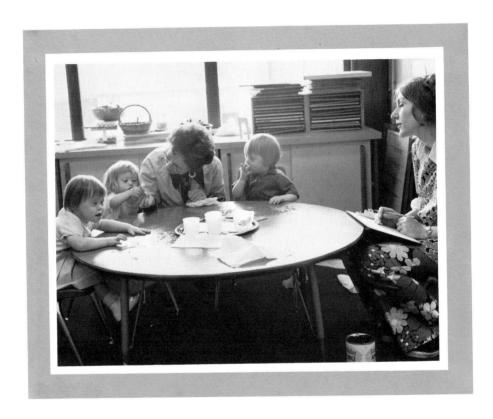

A time for juice and cookies provides a break in the class activities. The children, split into small groups, use this time to learn a few words, to sing songs together, and to develop their hand coordination. One teacher at each table records the children's progress.

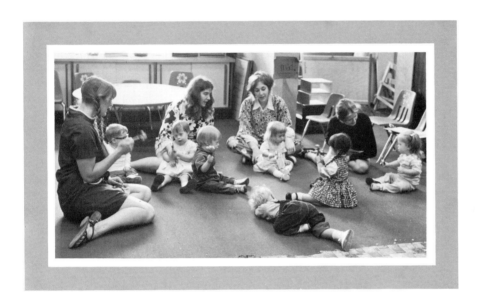

Near the end of every class is music time. There are bells and rhythm sticks to play in time to the piano. The children enjoy this "noisy" activity and it helps develop their sense of rhythm.

A DAY IN THE LIFE OF KENNY AT THE RAINIER STATE SCHOOL, BUCKLEY, WASHINGTON

Kenny is 14 years old, and lives in this attractive dormitory with about 200 other boys and girls in his age group. We visited Kenny on a lovely spring day and followed his activities from the moment he awoke in the morning until his picnic supper with the Boy Scouts that night. The Rainier State School is an excellent residence and school for the mentally deficient. It has spacious grounds and sits near the base of Mt. Rainier and the Cascade Mountain Range. Not all institutions are as attractive and provide as many educational, recreational, and social opportunities for their residents.

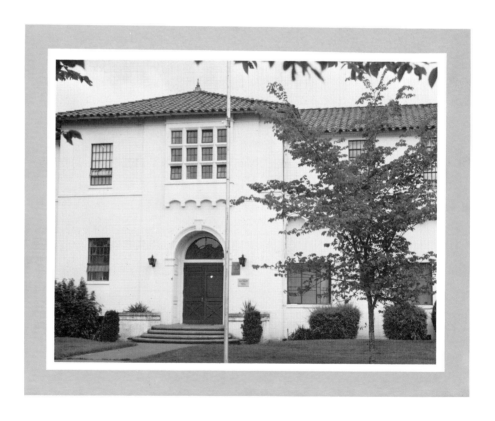

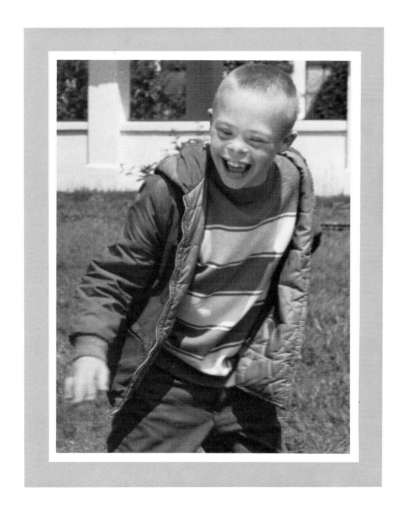

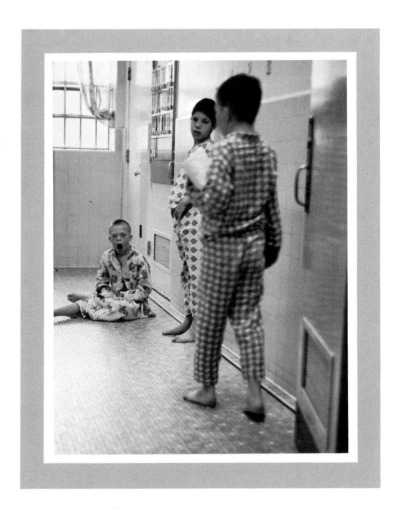

Like many kids, Kenny is a sleepyhead in the morning. He decides to relax a moment on the bathroom floor before brushing his teeth. At right, Kenny ponders over his breakfast cereal. The food at Rainier is good and plentiful, but a certain amount always seems to end up on the tablecloth and floor.

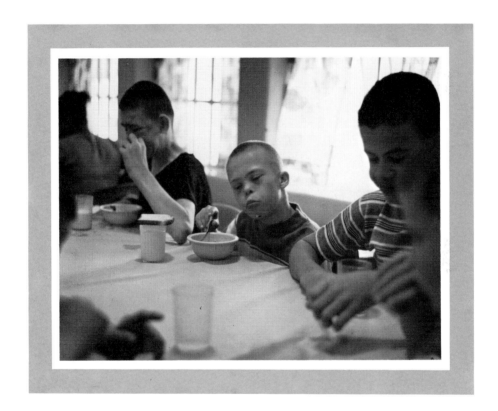

Kenny's intellectual level falls in the lower range for Down's syndrome children, and school is probably his least favorite part of the day. Below, he and his classmates are learning the letters of the alphabet. Every day there are also lots of songs to sing, games to play, and puzzles to fit together. These make learning arithmetic and word skills more enjoyable. Kenny loves to tie his shoelaces in knots. The teacher concentrates, at right, on unraveling the confusion. Kenny and a friend have a good romp outdoors after class. School ends at lunchtime, and the kids go back to their dormitories to eat and relax.

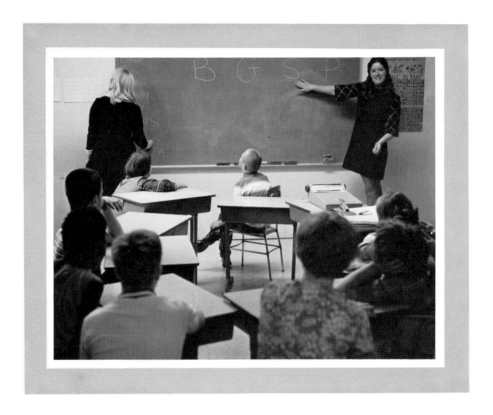

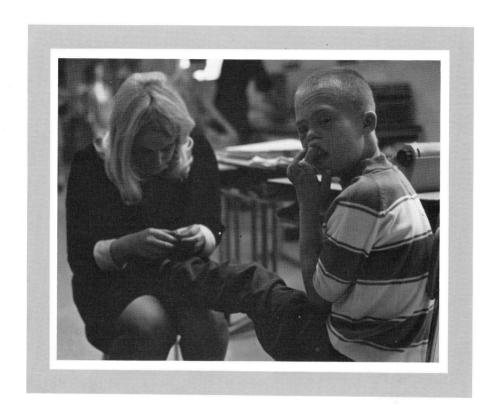

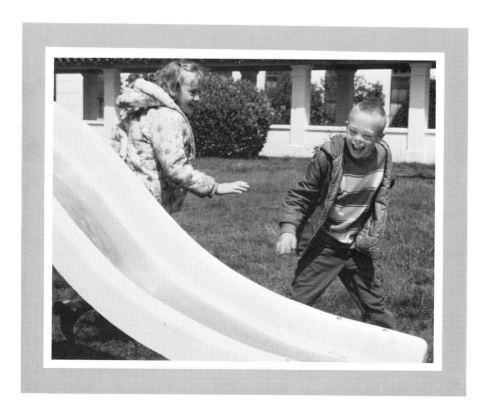

An hour's swim in the indoor pool is the highlight of Kenny's day. Being in the water is great fun for kids who can learn to swim and for those who are able simply to splash around and play. Most Down's syndrome children love the water and enjoy swimming at an early age.

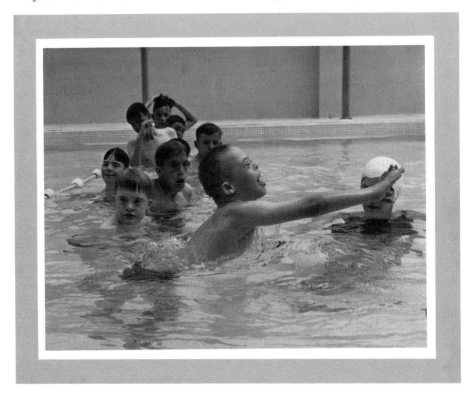

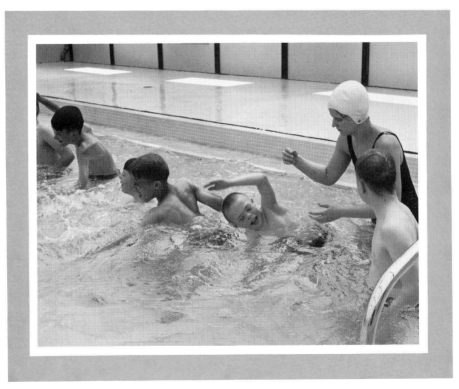

Several afternoons a week Kenny joins some of the other boys in the gym. There are a variety of activities to do to build coordination and balance, as well as confidence and courage. Down's syndrome children are often poorly coordinated, and these exercises help them perfect the simple skills of walking, running, and balancing. The trampoline is well suited to these purposes and great fun, too. It took Kenny a long time to muster up the courage to try the trampoline, and lots more to try some of the different jumps. Kenny's lack of good balance is a common characteristic of people with Down's syndrome.

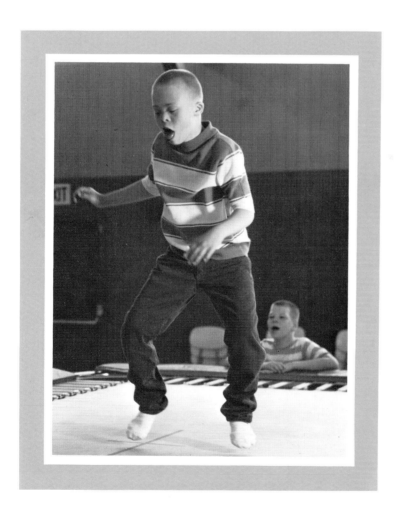

There are both Girl Scout and Boy Scout troops for the Rainier School residents. The Scouts schedule special activities and events that give the children a chance to go on outings and picnics. It's fun to dress up in a special shirt and kerchief and wear a Boy Scout cap and pin. At right, Kenny and his troop head off to the outlying areas of the School grounds where the picnic area is located. Below, one of the authors joins Kenny on his walk down the road. Kenny eagerly eats his supper after a long day of school and activities. At dusk the Scouts return to their dorms to play until bedtime.

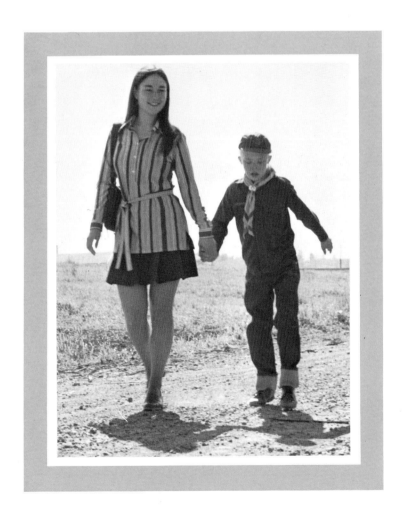

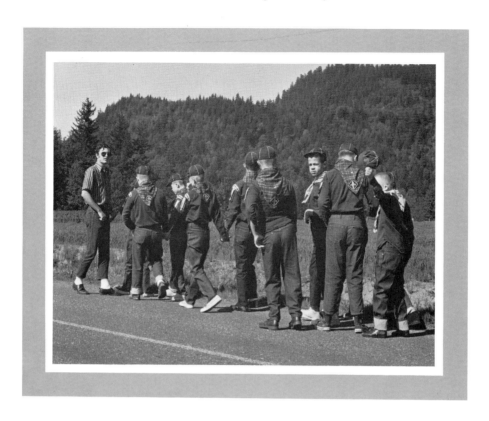

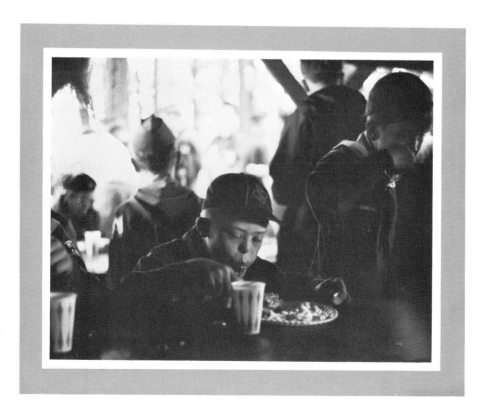

A VISIT WITH KATIE AND CAROLINE

Caroline, age 31, and Katie, age 54, live in a group home and go to work every day at a nearby sheltered workshop for mentally deficient people. For a long time both women were in an institution. Now, in middle age, they are discovering the satisfaction and fun that come from living in a family and doing something productive with their time each day. The group home is a busy, happy place. The "family" is composed of an energetic couple and their own youngsters plus several children with different mental and physical handicaps, and Caroline and Katie. The mother's sister and her husband and kids are frequent visitors around the house. An outdoor barbecue like the one shown here is usually a crowded, jolly affair where everyone mixes together, helping with supper, playing ball, and having a good time.

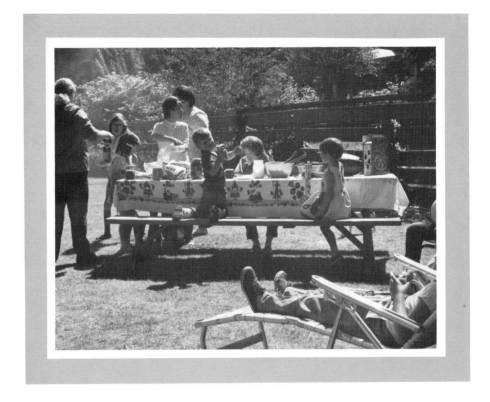

Katie and Caroline have certain chores around the house that they are expected to do. Everyone makes his own bed and tidies his room, as Caroline is doing. After dinner she puts the dishes in the dishwasher. Katie is very thorough with a broom, and can get the kitchen counters spotless with her sponge. All the members of the group home work together to keep things running smoothly and happily. Katie and Caroline seem to appreciate jobs they can be proud of.

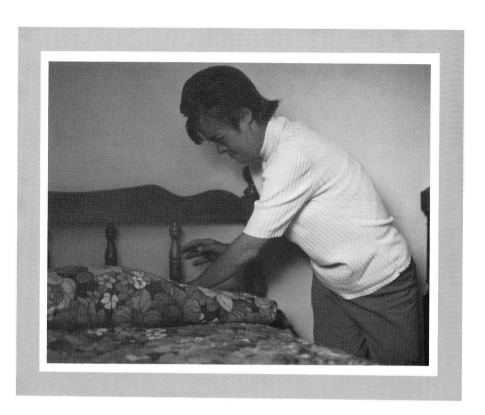

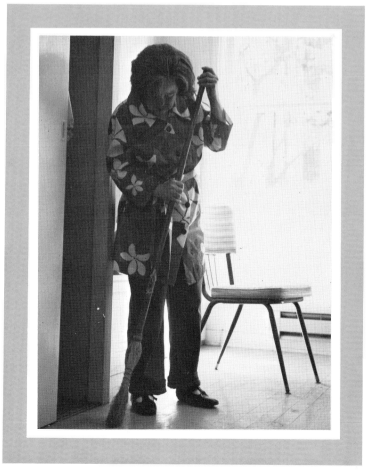

The house below is the sheltered workshop where Katie and Caroline work every day. The director, some assistants, and the mentally deficient who work there redid the old house and landscaped the yard. They laid pathways out and planted new trees, shrubs, and flowers. One of the director's many tasks is to find work from around the community for his people to do, often competing for small jobs with regular firms. Each person is then paid a certain amount for the work he does. Most of the people who come to the workshop have fairly limited abilities, so most jobs are fairly simple. The director has thought up a number of interesting projects to supplement the regular work activities. For example, the workshop members are hatching and raising quail, which are later sold to specialty food stores. Several summertime high school volunteers assist in the project. The director is a real farmer at heart, and has built a rabbit hutch in the yard. Caroline and the others get real pleasure out of caring for the animals. The money from the sale of the rabbits supplements the workshop's small income.

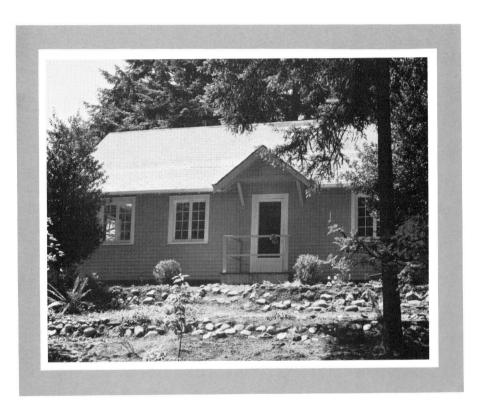

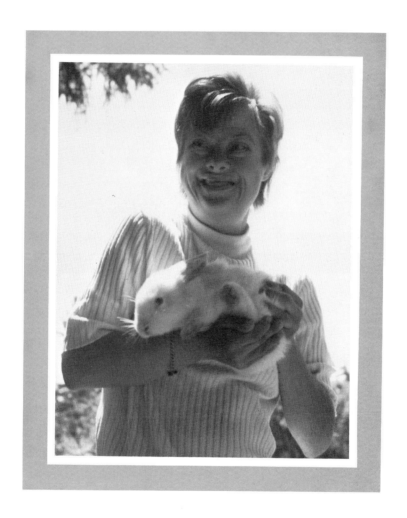

Inside the workshop are tables and chairs and a small kitchen. Here people work on their various projects. Caroline is sewing together net sponges to be sold. She is a good sewer and works very conscientiously. Katie, whose capabilities are fairly limited, enjoys the simple pleasures of coloring with crayons. As she gets older her eyesight is not as good. The workshop has a good-sized vegetable garden and orchard in the yard and Caroline seems to enjoy working outdoors. Many mentally deficient people receive a great deal of satisfaction working in simple agriculture, animal raising, and outdoor manual jobs.

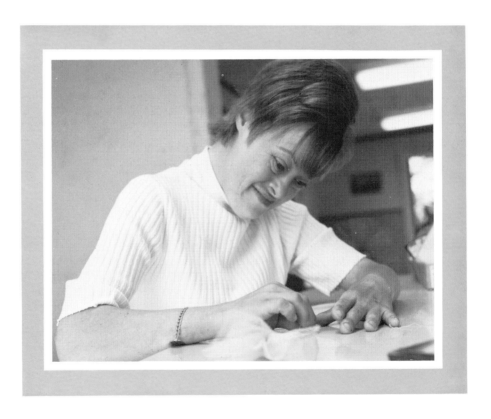

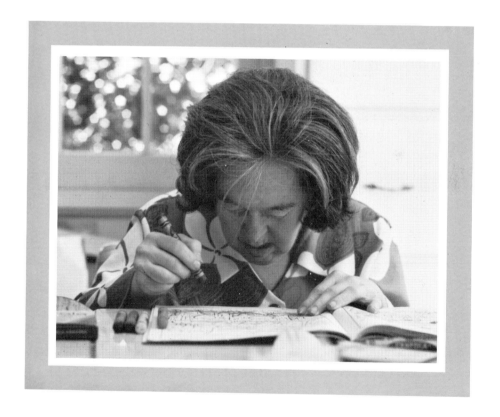

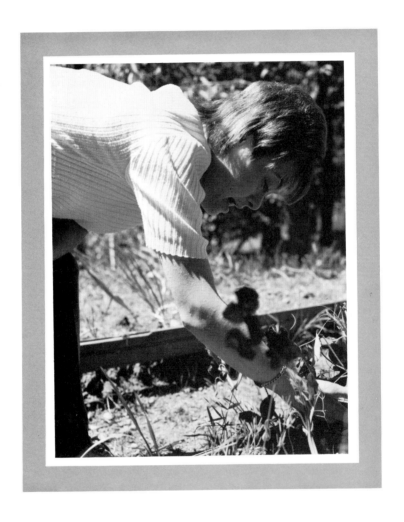

SOME OF THE OTHER FACES OF DOWN'S SYNDROME

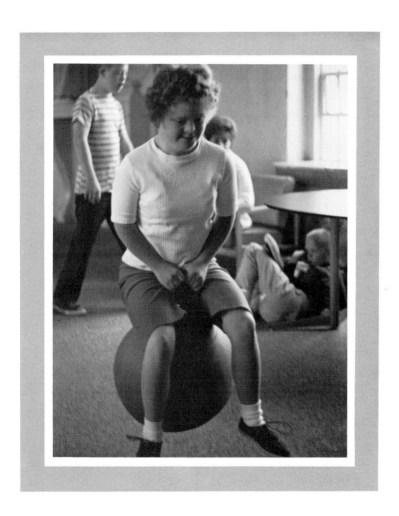

Bouncing a ball is not too much threat to the furniture in this big dormitory living room at the Rainier School.

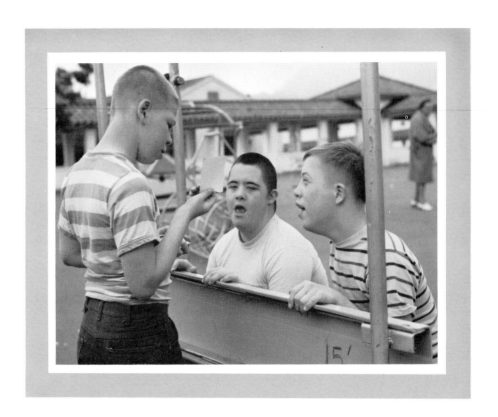

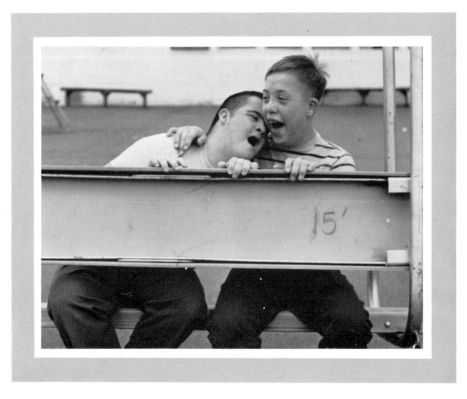

Three friends play school with homemade flashcards. They applaud themselves gleefully when they give a right answer.

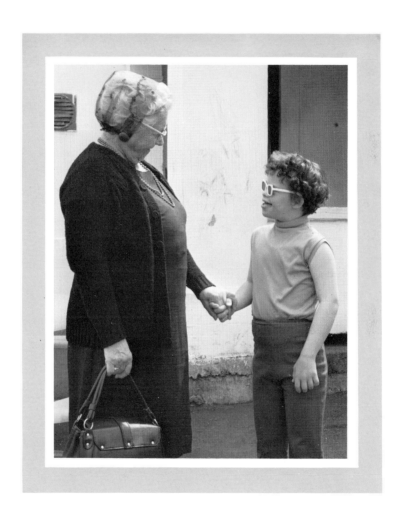

Older ladies in the community can be foster grandmothers at Rainier School. They visit their child regularly and go on walks, play games, or read together. This grandmother has brought her little girl a pair of green-tinted sunglasses as a gift, and received a hug as thanks.

Crossed eyes, as in this little girl on the left, are frequent in Down's syndrome youngsters, but may tend to go away gradually with time. Like the girl at the right, many of these need glasses.

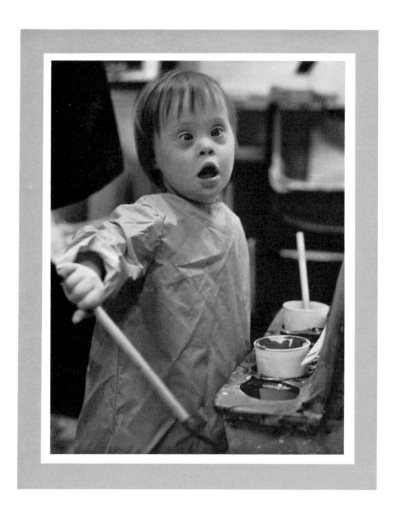

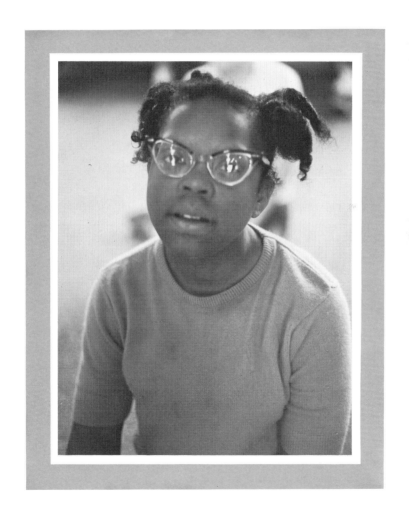

The Special Olympics for the Retarded are held every year in every state. There are usually local, state, and national meets, including competition in track, swimming, and other events. Usually the participants are students of the area's special school districts, residents of nearby institutions, and members of various recreational organizations for the mentally deficient. All the groups join in the parade around the University of Washington stadium where the Seattle Olympics are held. The little girl in the center carrying the banner has Down's syndrome. The fastest runner from last year's competition lights the eternal flame that burns throughout the meet. A young boy with Down's syndrome crosses the finish line, his chest already bedecked with ribbons.

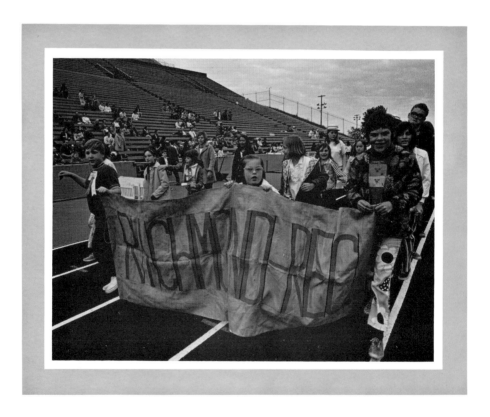

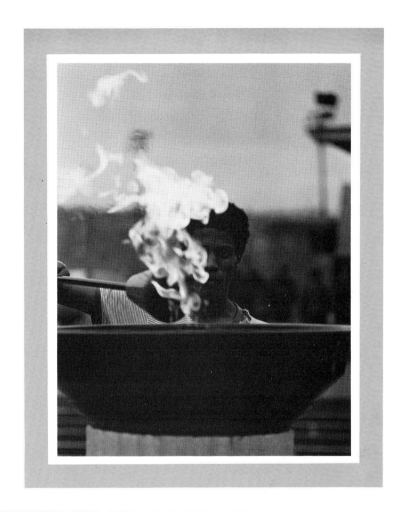

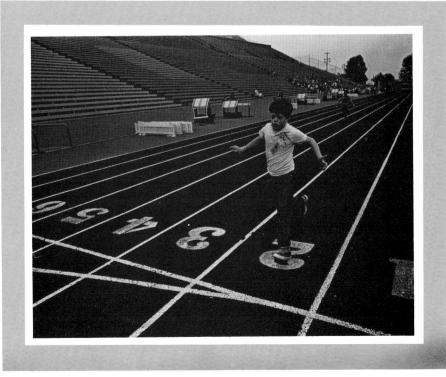

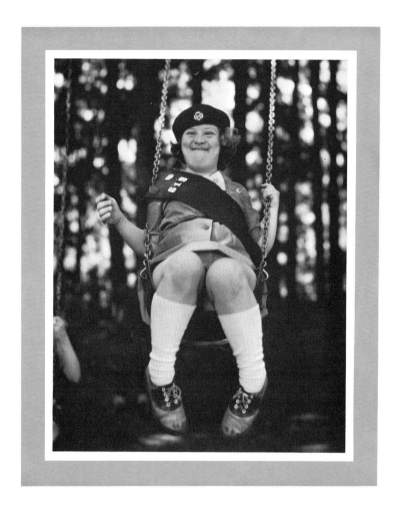

As they told you — we're happy people!

4

Adaptation of the Family and the Down's Syndrome Child

In this chapter, we are relating to parents observations derived from our own general experiences with families who have a child with Down's syndrome and presenting the statements from the parents of five children with Down's syndrome. We have learned that families vary greatly in their feelings about their child and his condition. Some of the thoughts expressed in this section may strike one person as true and meaningful, while to another person they may seem inappropriate or irrelevant. Our goal is to build a framework of ideas that may assist parents in formulating and understanding their own feelings and perspective. Many other people — doctors, relatives, friends — may contribute their thoughts. In the end, however, each parent determines his own feelings about his child and his role in the family. The process of adjusting to the birth of a child with limited potential is a uniquely personal thing. Some parents never adapt to it; others do so in remarkable fashion. There are no universal solutions or standards. Each family must find its own solution, and with time each one generally does.

Four Basic Thoughts in the Adjustment

There are four thoughts that we feel are important to keep in mind when adjusting to life with a Down's syndrome child. These ideas occur over and over again in this chapter and form the basis for most of what we say.

First, be honest about thoughts and emotions. Each parent must realistically confront his or her feelings about the child and his condition, and then be truthful and straightforward with the rest of the family. When there is a spirit of openness and concern, the best solution for everyone is more apt to be found.

Second, each member of the family is important and should be thought of and cared for. While the child with Down's syndrome may require a great deal of attention, understanding, and patience, he still is only one member of a group; in general, he should not take precedence over others, parents as well as children, in terms of love, attention, and understanding.

Third, the child with Down's syndrome can be loved and enjoyed as a real person. He can develop and express his own personality and feelings, and maintain his own special role as a member of a family or other group. Like everyone else, he should be encouraged and helped to develop to his own potential and to live a happy and satisfying life.

Lastly, the key to a wholesome situation for the family and the child is *acceptance* of the fact that the child has Down's syndrome and acceptance of the child himself. Acceptance, and to a certain extent approval, is necessary for the natural flow of affection, which in turn is necessary for the joy, warmth, and stimulation that parents and child derive from each other. Given acceptance, approval, and a natural flow of affection, there is seldom any problem for parents in the early rearing of a child with Down's syndrome. The baby is the guide; when he is ready and able to sit, walk, and talk he will do so; and when he is able to feed himself, be toilet-trained, and clothe himself it will usually become apparent with trials.

Without a realistic acceptance, there is serious risk of rejection or overprotection of the Down's syndrome child, either of which can have an adverse effect on the development of the child and on the family. There may be overexpectation or underexpectation for achievement, instead of stimulation of the child toward his *own* level of performance. Rejection can lead to chronic parental guilt feelings, and overprotection can be fed by unrealistic guilt feelings. Generally speaking, everyone loses when there is a lack of acceptance, and both the parents and the Down's syndrome child miss one of life's cherished phenomena, the natural flow of affection between parent and child.

Adjustment to the Baby with Down's Syndrome

When parents are told that their new baby has Down's syndrome, it is an unexpected shock. There may be a confusing jumble of events, feelings, and people. It usually takes a while before things begin to slow down and the reality of the situation becomes clear. In the first days, weeks, or even months after the baby's birth, some emotions and reactions may come and go rapidly, while others may remain constant. It is usually wise to remain flexible and not to make many permanent decisions in this early stage.

There is considerable variation among parents in the amount of time required for the process of coming to terms with the knowledge of a child's limited potential, and in the kind of emotional response involved in it. Many factors may play a role, such as a parent's past experience with mentally deficient children, or longstanding personal or family feelings about children and about abnormality, or the way in which the parent has learned to cope in the past with crises. Such experiences and feelings can sometimes make an initial adjustment to a Down's syndrome baby somewhat easier or more difficult. It is common for parents to feel a mixture of emotions and feelings such as disbelief, sadness, disappointment, anger, guilt, hope, curiosity, happiness. It is not unusual, too, for one parent to respond to the baby quite differently from the other. With different backgrounds and often different feelings about mental deficiency, a couple may need time to come to a common understanding and work out together a way of adapting to this unexpected situation. The early stages of adjustment may place a strain on the couple's marriage. Honesty and frankness with each other are important and necessary to insure that each person's feelings and desires are respected and considered. It seems a tragedy when the pressures of adjusting and living with a child with Down's syndrome go unresolved and are allowed to chip away at the strength and closeness of a marriage or a family.

Thoughts that May Help in the Initial Adjustment

There are two things parents can do to ease the process of getting to know and understand their new baby with Down's syndrome. The first is to learn what Down's syndrome is and how it alters a child's mental and physical development. The second is to spend time with the new baby, getting to know and enjoy him as he is. Of course, most babies don't show much social personality until they are about 2 to 3 months of age.

When the doctor first tells parents that their child has Down's syndrome, they are usually curious, and perhaps a little fearful, to learn how it is going to affect their child. It is to be hoped that the doctor will be able to provide up-to-date information about the condition, and will be gentle and flexible in his advice about the child's future. He may recommend that another doctor evaluate the baby or that the family visit a local mental retardation or congenital defects clinic that offers special services, such as chromosome studies, ongoing counseling, and later psychological testing. Regarding literature on Down's syndrome, most books published before 1962 will be inaccurate, at least in terms of the cause.

In most large communities there are chapters of the National Association for Retarded Children, and sometimes other organizations or parents' groups as well. From these local resources parents can obtain reading material and information about facilities in their area for services such as medical care, day care, and special education. The National Association for Retarded Children publishes a newsletter which includes news events concerning mentally deficient children, information about national and local programs, and reviews of new publications.

Perhaps the best way parents can learn about Down's syndrome and about life with a Down's syndrome child is to talk at length with parents who have had first-hand experience. A visit with a family that has an older child with Down's syndrome can show new parents not only what the growth and development of one child has been like, but also how one family has adapted to the problems and changes in their life style that have arisen throughout the years. Talking with several families whose Down's syndrome children are of different ages will give a broader picture of how various people have coped with a similar situation.

Equally important in the process of adjusting to the child with Down's syndrome is the time a parent spends becoming acquainted with the new baby. Concern for learning and understanding the facts about the condition can sometimes overshadow the importance of getting to know the baby as a real person with his own personality and characteristics. Ideally, both parents should make time to watch and hold and feed the baby. In the end, the best education comes from living with the Down's syndrome child and watching him grow up his own way, as he develops his personality and accomplishes what his potential allows.

Problems in the Initial Adjustment

First, it is usual for parents to anticipate that their child will be normal, and when they learn that the child has Down's syndrome they are often hurt and disappointed. The child who was born is not the child they were looking forward to, and they experience feelings of disbelief and then grief, almost as if the expected child had died. It takes a certain amount of time to accept the fact that the new baby will not be able to fulfill the expectations one has had for him, and then to formulate more realistic hopes for what he can do within the limits of his own potential. Until families can accept the limitations and alterations that Down's syndrome will place on their child, it will be difficult for them to accept and enjoy the child for what he is.

Second, some parents have difficulty working out a good relationship with their child's doctor. They may feel anger or resentment toward him after he tells them about the child's condition. This is a parental reaction that most doctors understand. It is always a difficult task to break "bad news" to people. Some doctors can do it sympathetically and with compassion; others are unable to. If parents are not satisfied with their doctor, they should find another one. A pediatrician who cares for Down's syndrome children and has knowledge of and experience with their problems may be helpful. But it is not wise to "switch" if you have faith and trust in your own doctor, for the care of a child with Down's syndrome does not differ appreciably from that of any other child.

Third, some parents find it difficult to tell their own parents, family members, and close friends about the baby's limited potential. In general, it is best to tell relatives simply and directly that the baby has Down's syndrome. Then they can be provided with information about what this will mean for the child as he grows up. Perhaps a doctor or counselor can speak with them if they have difficulty understanding it. It is best for parents to speak with them as soon as they themselves know about the condition and have begun to adjust to it. Often relatives and close friends can provide comfort and a new perspective to help parents in their adjustment. Occasionally, there is someone who cannot understand the situation from the parents' point of view and who forces his own feelings on them, causing anxiety and pain. If this happens, it is important for parents to remember that the baby is *their* child, and they alone must make the final decisions about what is best for him and their family. No one should be allowed to exert undue pressure or demands on parents when they are trying to find the best solution for the whole family.

Alternatives to Home Family Life for the Child with Down's Syndrome

Parents may wish to consider having the child with Down's syndrome live in an environment other than the family home. Such considerations should be frankly discussed with the doctor, who may ask the parents to consult with a social worker or other counselor. The following are some of the potential alternatives to living with the family. Such opportunities differ in both availability and quality among states and communities. However, the present tendency is toward enhancing the life situation for Down's syndrome children, both in the local communities and in the state institutions.

PART-TIME

Early Age: Day care centers; special pre-school programs.

Mid-childhood and Later: Special education programs in public schools; sheltered workshops for limited training and jobs (rare today).

FULL-TIME

Foster Home: When early placement outside the home is indicated, it is usually to a foster home. The foster mother, who generally is paid by the state, is often a dedicated woman who provides good mothering and care.

Institutions for the Mentally Deficient: Most state institutions will not accept infants and very young children with Down's syndrome because of a lack of facilities plus the conviction that they cannot provide adequate "mothering" in the more crucial early years of a child with Down's syndrome. Admission policies vary, as does the quality of the life situation and training programs in such institutions, which are most commonly called training schools. Parents should become acquainted with the nature of their state's institution(s). Some are ideal and provide a better environment and training situation for the Down's syndrome child than could be found in the average home and community. Others are predominantly custodial in nature.

The basic decision regarding institutional care and training is left strictly with the parents. Parents may wish to consider some of the following thoughts in their own deliberations about institutional care and training:

1. When the child with Down's syndrome reaches the age of 4 to 6 years, it becomes rather difficult for him to find appropriate playmates—a peer group—in the home situation. About 20 per cent of the residents of institutions for the mentally deficient have Down's syndrome. These people usually enjoy each other's company, are clannish, and help each other.

2. In general, the social situation and the training programs in the in-

stitutions are geared for persons with Down's syndrome, and the personnel understand them. Those with Down's syndrome who are able to work can perform jobs at the institution or, occasionally, part-time jobs in a nearby community. They usually come to feel "at home" and, with rare exception, are happy in an institution.

3. The adjustment to life in an institution may be easier and more complete following admission at the age of 5 to 10 years than at 15 to 20 years.

4. The person with Down's syndrome will probably never be able to function as an independent adult, and hence will always be dependent on someone.

5. Most institutions allow frequent visiting and short- or long-term home leaves, according to the parents' wishes.

Group Home: A rather new development is that of smaller group homes for the moderately mentally deficient within the community, usually run by a family. These homes may be affiliated with a community sheltered workshop, allowing for limited job opportunities.

THE PERSONAL EXPERIENCE AND COMMENTS OF PARENTS

The following are the unedited statements from members of five families who kindly consented to share their experience with their child with Down's syndrome and give counsel to other parents. The authors were not involved in the diagnosis or counsel in all of these cases. The parents were asked to comment on the following: (1) their family situation at the time of birth of the Down's syndrome baby; (2) their initial response when they were told their child had Down's syndrome; (3) their child's story and any problems they have had; and (4) a few recommendations for new parents of a child with Down's syndrome.

ROBERT, 14 WEEKS OLD

We are both 30 years old and are in the middle income bracket. I am a full-time mother, as we have two other boys in addition to Robert who is 14 weeks old.

When Robert was born he appeared to us to be as normal as any newborn baby. He was a big baby of 8 pounds 1 ounce. Our pediatrician came the morning after he was born and broke the news. He tried to explain that Robert had an extra set of chromosomes which causes a serious problem. I was so shocked that what he had to say did not really register. I called my husband and tried to explain that we were going to have problems with Robert. He tried to settle me down but it was of no avail. After that I was too upset to take the baby. Later in the day I walked down to the nursery to see the baby, and it was still hard to believe anything was wrong.

That afternoon Bob and a couple of relatives came to visit. They settled me down. They could not see anything wrong, either. About this time the baby developed yellow jaundice which we thought was probably normal. But the doctor feared that it might be a complication. The week after taking the baby home our doctor made arrangements to take Robert to a clinic where a group of doctors could examine him and confirm his diagnosis.

We did this when Robert was about 2 weeks old. Once again we were told that he had Down's syndrome and what caused it. We were also told some of the things to expect. This again was very hard to take.

Bob got some advice from his boss, who has a 21-year-old daughter with cerebral palsy. The advice he gave was get expert professional help immediately and do not take what the doctors have to say for granted. A group of doctors had told him his daughter would never walk or talk. She now walks with the help of braces and talks plainly. Robert is now 14 weeks old and is an extremely happy baby. We enjoy him so much. We anticipate every advancement he makes. He started rolling over when he was 5 weeks old and started creeping at 8 weeks. We are very pleased with the help we are getting from many professional people in our community which includes therapy for his physical development and help from a nutritionist in an attempt to keep his weight and height in proportion.

For new parents of a newborn child with Down's syndrome, treat him like you would a normal child. Give him the same love and attention you would give a normal child. Probably it is best not to give him any more attention than you give any of your other children. Do not let the child be your entire life. It is not fair to the rest of your family. We look upon Robert the same as our other boys, but as one who needs a little more help in developing. We are fortunate to live in a school district that has a special school for these children. It is a new school but we understand the results have been outstanding to date. The important thing is not to get discouraged, as more and more is being developed in the line of learning aids for this special child.

B.J., 3 YEARS OLD

When I found out at 44 years of age that I was pregnant I imagine that my husband and I were about the happiest couple in the world. We already had two sons, 15 and 13, but had wanted another child and had never taken any steps to prevent having one.

My husband has his own business and is well established and our sons are good students and happy in our home. We have what we feel is an extremely good and healthy relationship with the boys and are very proud of both of them. I had a wonderful full-term pregnancy and our sons were as happy as my husband and I.

It was a very few hours after my baby was born that our pediatrician came to my room and told me that our baby girl was retarded. At that moment the bottom dropped out of my whole world and I wished that both the baby and I could die right there.

When we brought the baby home I shed many tears in the quiet of the night and had thoughts that even my husband never knew about.

But now, 3½ years later, I ask myself, "What was it—sorrow for the baby or sorrow for myself?"

This dear child is the joy of our life.

When the sorrow passes, and believe me it does, then the happiness sets in. Every moment of every day is a complete revelation of what these children can do and accomplish.

Our daughter was completely trained for the toilet when she was 2½ years of age. She tries to dress herself and eats beautifully with a fork and on her own initiative is learning to use her knife properly.

When she was 1½ years of age I decided that she was doing so well, but even with the love that she was surrounded with, there had to be more to her life. I took it upon myself to phone the University of Washington, which I had read had started a new Developmental Center.

Within 3 weeks, my husband and I had an appointment.

They started our daughter in a beginning nursery program and a year later had her start in a new program strictly for Down's syndrome children. This was just like regular kindergarten.

It is unbelievable what they have done with these children.

We know that our daughter is not going to go to a university or anywhere near it, but she will do her own thing and will become independent to a degree, and in the meantime to see her progress as she has has been an answer to all our prayers.

Her comprehension is well above normal, which makes it easier because she understands everything we say to her. She is a bit slow in speech, but they have already started her in beginning speech therapy. Even at 3 she is small for her age, but a lovely looking child. Her attention span is quite remarkable, and needless to say we love her dearly — not because we feel sorry for her, but because she *is* such a *special* child.

As to the future for B.J., I really don't look that far ahead. We take each day as it comes.

Financially she will be taken care of, and I have a dream that some day when B.J. and her friends at the University are older there will be a type of group home for older Down's syndrome young adults. Not an institution-type school, but a loving home that they could come home to after doing some type of work they had been trained for.

Of course this would be if something happened to my husband and me, because we hope to have her with us always.

For new parents of a Down's syndrome baby, I feel that the sooner you can be in touch with other parents of such children the better. Even to have these parents visit you in the hospital. Visit these children in school, etc., and you will find your whole outlook will change. You will no longer have this feeling that you are the only parents that this ever happened to, and all that loneliness will disappear.

As early as possible get your youngster into a special education program. You will be amazed at what these children can learn and thrilled at what they can accomplish.

Most of all, love them dearly and you will find it is returned to you tenfold. From my heart I can truthfully say, everyone should be so blessed.

SANDRA, 15 YEARS OLD, RAISED AT HOME TILL 8 YEARS OLD

In the year 1957, May 15th, our family had four members in it. Mother, Virginia, age 26; father, Gene, age 31, a television technician repairman; and two sons, Scott, 3½ years old, and Steve, 8 years old. We were anxiously awaiting the arrival of our new baby. My husband and I had been dreaming about the little girl we were at least hopeful of having.

Gene even went so far as to buy a sewing machine for me to fashion little dresses for her.

The evening of May 15th I started preparing dinner and it was made obvious the time was near for our new arrival to make an appearance into the world. Within an hour I was in hard labor. We didn't finish dinner, things happened too fast.

Sandra Jean was born at 8:45, 15 minutes after we arrived at the hospital. I was wide awake. It was just too wonderful to be true, I really had a little girl. What a wonderful beautiful world!

Gene wasn't so lucky to live in this happy atmosphere. The doctor told him something was wrong. The baby hadn't responded normally. She was too passive. Healthy yes, but just too content. Gene was asked to ask our pediatrician to consult with our obstetrician.

The next morning the two doctors confirmed that our baby was a mongoloid child. Up to this time I knew nothing about this. I had been in heaven all night thinking about my beautiful little girl. Even when I slept I dreamed of her.

Three times during the night I asked the nurse to please get my baby, undress her and let me see for myself if I really, truly had given birth to a little girl.

Well, my bliss ended about 9:00 A.M. The pediatrician who had made the diagnosis came to my room and broke the news. This in itself seemed cruel. Why didn't he call my husband so we could be together when told? He explained to me what a mongoloid child was. He advised against us even taking her home. He said it would be a mistake to become attached to her. She would be a burden, little mental progress could be expected, and we would only have heartache after heartache. Financially we couldn't afford having someone else to care for her; besides, this would be the last thing in the world I could do. You don't start loving a child after birth; my child had been loved from the moment I knew I was pregnant. As she started moving about in the womb this love increased.

The hospital was very kind. The staff knew I was in a state of shock, not knowing how to handle our new situation. They did everything to make me comfortable. When I came home I was in a deep depression. For a while the future looked so bleak, I thought perhaps it might be best to take my life along with my child's. I had been led to believe there was no future with this child. My mind was so mixed up I couldn't think straight. I did my housework and cared for my family in a daze.

Every time I took Sandra in for a checkup, I was hoping I had been dreaming and the doctor would announce there had been a mistake, my child was perfectly normal. This never happened. Instead, he made it clear even the progress I told him about probably was an exaggeration on my part. He or the nurse would tell me I should get pregnant again as soon as possible. Even God makes mistakes and my child was one of them. I was told that I must accept this. Well I don't believe this, I think my child is a very special person, she deserves to be cared for just like any child.

As Sandra began to grow and develop we found she was a very affectionate child. Her love for our family and people she came in contact with was endless. Sandra loves everyone.

Steve and Scott played with Sandra a lot. They loved to wrestle with her and she had a wonderful time with them.

Sandra was never allowed to lie idle. I picked her up out of the crib as she awoke. I spent a lot of time massaging her legs and arms to build up her muscle tone.

At about 7 months we changed pediatricians. The new doctor told us to take Sandra home and love her, not to try to solve all problems. She needed to be trained and above all loved.

This was the turning point in our thinking, just knowing someone approved of the love we had for Sandra and the desire to keep her with us.

Sandra's development was really quite good. She was energetic, inquisitive and always laughing. At 7 months she was rolling all over the house and not long after, crawling very well. She sat alone at 9 months. At 13 months she could stand and walk holding on to things, such as the coffee table. She walked alone 2 weeks before her second birthday, and, I might add, like an expert. The only fear she had in walking was stairs; even now she holds on tight to the bannister. Sandra was completely potty-trained at 2½ years.

The fall after her second birthday, Mrs. Beryl Gridley, the principal of Woodside School (a school for the handicapped) offered me and several other parents of retarded children the basement of her home to have a play group for our children in. This and our joining the Washington Association for Retarded Children was the true beginning of our accepting Sandra for what she is. No more, no less. We wanted to be sure she had every chance to become her full potential as a human being. I truly believe she is a very special child, not a mistake of God's.

If only all parents of a mongoloid child could be told what a blessing in so many ways their child could be instead of what a burden and all the problems after problems they could expect, maybe they wouldn't have to go through the fear we did.

Up until Sandra was 5 years old I was actively engaged in working with my retarded child and others in the community. In February of 1962 I became pregnant and had to quit working. My pregnancy went along fine except it was very hard for me to find time to rest. Sandra no longer took naps in the daytime.

October 2nd, 1962, we had our second little girl, Kelly Marie. Of course we lived in fear the whole 9 months of pregnancy, but Kelly is healthy and normal in every way. She progressed so much faster than Sandra did. Sandra enjoyed having a little sister and was very kind to her.

There are hard parts of raising a child like this that aren't easy, but with the right perspective they don't seem nearly so bad. The fact that Sandra was hyperactive tried my energy to no end. I think the hardest part of caring for Sandra was the fact she knew no fear of other people. We couldn't keep her in our fenced yard, she always found a way out. If she heard a noise she was off to find where it came from. She was lost in the neighborhood many times. Also, children in the neighborhood were not very kind to her. I guess they found it hard to cope with her inability to talk plainly. They tired of her quickly, leaving Sandra still wanting to play more, but with no one to play with. Then we had a lot of tears. This broke my heart. Also, many mothers didn't want Sandra to play with their children for fear she would hurt them. Sandra is and always was a gentle person, but when pushed can become very stubborn. Of course, being larger and older in years than the children who played at her level made it difficult. This is where play group and school with children like her or with similar problems seemed to be the answer.

At 8 years of age we admitted Sandra to Rainier School (a state institution for the mentally deficient). Not because we don't love her, but because we care too much to see her at home with no playmates and idle. What the future has in store for our special child I don't know. Maybe when she reaches maturity we will again have her home. This depends on Sandy's happiness and family circumstances.

Right now Sandra is a very happy child. She received an award for excellent behavior at school; also, she is in their Girl Scout program and marches with their drill team. Sandra is capable of complete self-help and does a nice job of self-grooming. She likes her hair short and lets me know when it is time for a haircut. Sandra learned to swim a little this last summer and can turn somersaults in the water. We have her home on weekends as often as possible and on all holidays.

I think the first advice I would give to a parent of a newborn mongoloid child would be to love the child for what he is. Not to try and solve everything at once. Second, seek expert advice. Go to the Association for Retarded Children and meet other parents with problems similar if not worse than your own.

I can't say we are always happy with our situation. Sometimes we feel guilt in not having her home all the time. But then we have to remind ourselves how happy Sandra is. We at this time couldn't give her the well rounded experiences she has at Rainier School.

Having Sandra for a child has taught us compassion, humbleness, and true love for our fellow man. God has been good to us and I hope we never become too proud to appreciate what we have.

A very special person in our lives, my stepmother, wrote this poem about our special child. We would like to share it with you.

SANDY
We have a lovely Angel
God sent her down one day
I guess he thought we needed her
That's why he let her stay.
She's such a lovely angel
And I hope that folks will understand
And if her steps should falter
They'd stop and lend a hand.
I don't know why she came to us
It's not ours to question why.
This lovely Angel from on high
I've seen her grow so proudly
Sheltered by those tender arms
Keeping watch their silent vigil
Shielding her from danger's harm.
We know this little Angel
Is such a special one
And we will guard her fiercely
Each and every one.
We don't know if this precious child
Is with us here to stay
I only know we'd miss her
If she ever went away.
Tho doubts and fears assail us
We'll walk along in faith
Knowing well no other one
Could ever take her place.

Ruth Grissom

KENNY, 15 YEARS OLD, RAISED AT HOME TILL 8 YEARS

Kenny's Mother: I was born and raised in a small town. I came from a family of three children and am an identical twin. I completed high school and worked a couple of years in a restaurant and a department store and helped put my husband through college, which he didn't quite complete, plus being a homemaker for our five children.

Shortly after we were married I had a major operation which consisted of removal of one ovary and part of another. My organs were in the wrong place. I had a growth and several cysts and my appendix removed.

Kenny, our first-born child, a mongoloid son, came real early—I would guess 2 months early. All through my pregnancy with Kenny I had severe back problems. I can't ever remember when I did anything while I carried him—the pains in my back never let up. The doctor gave me shots two and three times a week. He said it was the ligaments in my back which would spread out and not go back into shape. When he gave me the shots I would pass out and my husband would carry me out to the car. What kind of shots I don't know. I was turned over to another doctor, a baby doctor, who delivered our son. Kenny was breech and was blue in color when he was born. He had all the symptoms of a mongoloid but I didn't know that. Looking back now, I know. I asked the doctor who delivered him about his color and he said he was a normal premature baby. My mother made the comment that she had twins that were premature and they never looked like her grandson.

We found out about Kenny after our second child was born. Kenny was about 14 months old when he started to go backwards. Words that meant something to him had no meaning anymore. His speech and coordination were poor, he developed colds continually, and he didn't walk until he was 3 years old. Everything came slow to our son. As parents we began to wonder what was wrong but the doctor kept telling us he was premature and they are slower. He always found an excuse. Finally my husband told me to take our son to another doctor who knows us as a family and find out what was wrong. I went with my husband's folks and took our son in. The doctor took one look at me and asked who was with me, or was I alone. I told him I came with the grandparents. He then said, come into my office. I followed and sat down with Kenny. He looked me straight in the face and said your son is retarded and I suggest you put his name and application into Rainier School as soon as possible before there is too long a waiting list. He said something might happen to me or my husband and we had our other child to think of. When I left the office the tears came. I couldn't think of a thing, I was so upset and shocked and numb and hurt and maybe even bitter because it had happened. I even wondered why it had to be us. What wrong did we do? My husband's folks told Lloyd. I'll never forget the hurt, but my husband is one who always makes and accepts the problem regardless of what it is. Time has passed now but I can always see and feel the hurt in my husband. I love Kenny, and he will always have a special place in my heart, but if he was at home all the time my love would change and I never would want that. Kenny is very hard to handle and with four other children I couldn't do it. He is so active and into everything from morning till night.

We put Kenny into Rainier School when he was 8 years old. We had

10 days to accept or refuse. The days just flew by. This was one of the hardest decisions in our lives. I just didn't know, and my husband wouldn't say, so I took it on myself and went to his doctors and his school-teachers to find out his abilities and his progress, which was slow. I transported Kenny to school for 3 years because there were no facilities in our area for the retarded. I had a feeling of trying to give him as much opportunity as possible. After talking to the doctors, teachers, and personal friends plus relatives I found that the recommendations conflicted. My husband's folks said no. My folks said yes. I decided only my husband and I could find the answer. Again I talked to my husband. The deadline was near. He just couldn't give me an answer. I know this will sound silly and I'm not a religious person, but there is a time you need help. I think I prayed harder then to find an answer. All of a sudden I looked at myself as a wife and mother with the responsibility of the other four children. I felt that with Kenny being home I would fail in my other duties. Kenny is very retarded — he must be continually watched. When a person gets older, as Kenny gets older, I know deep in my heart I couldn't handle him anymore. This I know I would have to accept because it existed. For the future there is little hope for Kenny but research will come up with something and there's always hope that something will develop in the future.

Kenny's father: I am the father of Kenny. I am now 41 years old. I was 26 when Ken was born. My wife was 22.

I was born and raised along with an identical twin brother on a pretty much average dairy and beef farm in western Washington. I completed grade school, high school, and 3½ years of college. My home community is small. The town has a population of about 400 with a large rural population. High school had an enrollment of about 150 in those days. It now has 300. I was very active in school and community activities. I have worked in plywood mills, logging camps, on construction jobs, and in creameries to get through school. However, I never have gotten the desire to farm out of my blood.

After getting married I decided to return to college, majoring in Animal Science. I thought this would be one way of staying close to farming but still getting away from the long 16-hour day. I thought it would also be more rewarding financially. During our third year at school we encountered many medical expenses without any insurance to help.

At this point graduates in this field were leaving school to take jobs of less than $4,000. An opening had now come up at home in the local Post Office. I had applied many years before and had nearly forgotten about it. The salary was not anything spectacular but I knew the job would be steady. We had many doctor bills. There was no way to return to school and get my degree. Besides, our first child was on its way. After only a very little thought we decided to take the job. I reasoned that I could start here and get started part-time farming, which we did. I had had my fill of apartment living by this time and was going to raise my family in a rural community.

After 8 months of a terribly complicated pregnancy and nearly 2 weeks of "on and off" (mostly on) labor, our first child was born.

At this time I did not know that he was to be retarded — a child with Down's syndrome. He was premature, his complexion was almost a blackish blue, and of course he had the features of the mongoloid. These I did not recognize, as I had never seen such a youngster before. Besides, he was the first child, a boy at that. His condition was very critical and with all the hopes and plans there were for him we could only think of saving him. I could not have dreamed of anything else. My mother-in-law was with me. She knew immediately that something was not right and asked the doctor what was wrong. We were told the youngster was premature. She told the doctor she knew better, as she had herself had two premature babies, neither of which looked like this.

After nearly a month in the hospital and after several days of instruction on how to feed a baby whose reflexes had not developed we were able to bring him home for Christmas.

We were so proud of him. My folks, who at this time had only granddaughters, were also happy for he was their first grandson. I could see Dad's eyes light up—I knew he could almost see Ken roping the calves, breaking that calf, driving the tractor and truck, helping to put up the hay, and all that goes with this business of farming.

Yes, by now we had made the down payment on a little farm where we were living. This was just a stepping stone to something larger. Lots of big plans for the little guy.

But "Kenny" was so slow. When asked why, the doctor said: "He's a preemie." This excuse eventually wore out. He did not walk, he did not talk, and after 14 months started to go backward. Words which once had a meaning and were associated with things now were just words. Other friends had preemies but they progressed much faster. At 32 months he took his first step. One whose youngster walked at 6 to 12 months could never have been so excited. At 36 months he started to walk. His 2-years-younger sister walked at nine months.

We became more concerned. Now we knew, everyone else knew, but no one would say anything. After all, I guess, how could they?

When the local doctor told us, it was the hardest day of my life. Yes, deep down inside I knew, but I really didn't want to know it. It was a bitter pill to take. No one wants to accept this kind of fact. Besides there were too many hopes and plans which this didn't fit into.

Finally I realized that if we were to help ourselves and Kenny we would have to accept the fact and go on from there doing whatever could be done to help him.

First, he would not be able to get to a regular public school. There were no facilities and besides, his coordination was too poor for him to get around with other children.

Kenny was always joyful and happy and so lovable—very affectionate. However, he would on occasions be harmful to the other smaller youngsters. He could not be left with the other babies. You had to keep an eye on him every minute. As the younger children progressed past him he became more frustrated and living together became much more trying for everyone. He would often times pick up toys, etc., and hit the smaller children, not realizing what damage he could do.

He was to have three sisters and one brother, all younger than him. Birthdays were 2 to 3 years apart. As each youngster passed him by physically and mentally he would then play with the next younger, all the while becoming more frustrated.

After transporting him 45 miles a day for special schooling and after counseling with doctors and teachers we decided to make application for his admittance to Rainier School.

Many were the heartaches for everyone. But as the heartaches grew so did the will and determination to fight for this youngster. He could not defend himself so we all found ourselves trying to protect him.

At 8 years of age, the last of November, we were informed that there was an opening at Rainier School. We had 10 days to accept or reject. The thought of not having him home for Christmas I hated to think of. His mother now had four other smaller youngsters to care for. She had transported him 5 days a week to school, driving 45 miles for 3 years. He had become harder to handle and there were more problems between the youngsters. We knew that we could not go on this way much longer. Reluctantly I consented to take a tour of the school. Seeing that he would have 24-hour-a-day care, there was only one decision we could come to. We knew we could not give him this type of care and training at home. Although we knew it was the right thing, this no doubt was the hardest decision of our lives. No one else could have made it. It had to be us. Kenny would go away to school.

Now, looking back after 15 years, I see it was the right thing to do. Kenny comes home for holidays, his birthday, and vacations. We love him as always, probably more than if we had had to live together all the time.

If I were to give advice to a new parent of a child with Down's syndrome, I think I would first say: "Thank God it happened today," for these children now are accepted by society. Not many years ago this was not so. The training and schooling available is remarkable.

Don't ever think your love will be less for this youngster. Believe me, this child will always have an extra special place in your heart. Yes, of course, you have been hurt. You feel the whole world has fallen on you. No, it need not be so. You now have a great challenge before you. You will also find new and added strength to fight for yourself and family. Be ever so grateful for the facilities that we have. Society now accepts these youngsters for what they are.

We have four perfectly normal youngsters, all born after this youngster. Our second was not planned — we were both scared to death. We didn't need to be. Thank God for such an accident, for we now have a family which otherwise we would not have dared to have.

My family and I have been active in community and social activities. We are just as well accepted now as we were before. We have now had the opportunity to show others what these youngsters can do and that they can reward you as a parent in their way. First thing, however, and above all, you must accept the fact that your youngster is what he is, so you can then face the problem straight on. You can now help both yourself and the youngster. Don't stop now to feel sorry for yourself. You have lots of company and what we do can be a lesson to those who follow us. Don't be ashamed, for you need not be. Lift your head up high, dry those tears, and start to fight, for there is much work to be done.

A BABY WHO DID NOT SURVIVE, BECAUSE OF A HEART DEFECT

At the time our child was born, my husband and I were both 38 years old. We had three healthy teen-age sons, and we were all delighted with the thoughts of having a baby in the house.

Throughout my pregnancy, I was plagued by severe edema and activation of a heart murmur, things which had not troubled me in the previous pregnancies. So I felt much relief when I first saw our baby, who looked so healthy and well formed, although much smaller than the others (5 pounds to their 8 pounds).

But our relief was short-lived. Almost immediately he began having respiratory problems, and his vital organs (heart) did not function properly. I was worried that my problems were to blame, but the doctors ruled this out. For one terrible week he battled for life, but they were unable to save him.

It was not until after the autopsy that we learned he had Down's syndrome. We were already in a state of shock, great disappointment, and sorrow. In our case, the fact that he had Down's syndrome helped us to better accept his death as a merciful act of God — because, with his lack of oxygen, he would have had extensive brain damage, and probably no chance of any normal life.

To other parents, we can only recommend the following: (1) do not indulge in self-pity; (2) become as informed as possible on this handicap — knowledge is essential in adapting your lives to this situation; and (3) support and have faith in medical research, your child, and God.

REFERENCES

The following are a few references to articles or books written by parents of Down's syndrome children; the last is written by an unusual man with Down's syndrome.

Hayakawa, S. J.: Our son, Mark. *McCall's Magazine* 97:78–9, Dec. 1969.

Roberts, Mr. and Mrs. Bruce: *David*. 1968. John Knox Publisher, Box 1176, Richmond, Va. 23209.

Hunt, N.: *The World of Nigel Hunt: The Diary of a Mongoloid Youth*. 1967. Garrett Publications, 29 West 57th St., New York, N.Y. 10019.